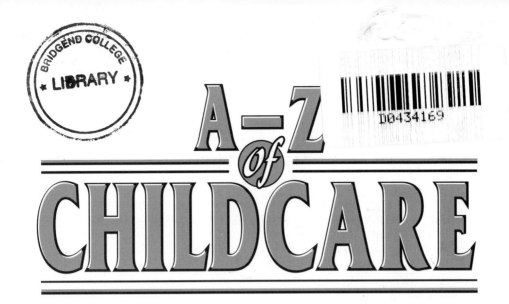

A–Z of CHILDCARE

THE COMPLETE STUDY GUIDE AND PROJECT PLANNER

Christine Hobart • Jill Frankel

STANLEY THORNES (PUBLISHERS) LTD

First published in 1998 by
Stanley Thornes (Publishers) Ltd
Ellenborough House
Wellington Street
CHELTENHAM
Glos GL50 1YW
UK

98 99 00 01 02 / 10 9 8 7 6 5 4 3 2 1

A catalogue record for this book is available from the British Library.

ISBN 0-7487-3189-X

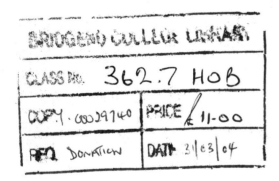
Typeset by Columns Design Ltd, Reading
Printed and bound in Great Britain by Redwood Books, Trowbridge, Wiltshire

CONTENTS

ACKNOWLEDGEMENTS

We would like to thank our colleagues, past and present, at City and Islington College for their continued support and encouragement.

A special thank you goes to Liza Martello for suggesting that we write this book, and to Zoe Halfon for the 'General Essay Plan' on page 16.

Thank you also to Marion Beaver et al for the use of Appendix B, and to CACHE for the use of Appendix C.

HOW TO USE THIS BOOK

Your ability to succeed on any course of study, increase your self-confidence and develop a professional attitude will depend on your ability to study, carry out research and apply this knowledge to your practical skills. The aim of this book is to help you develop these skills and build your knowledge.

The book is divided into three parts, each with a unique purpose, but each linking with the others.

Study skills

The study skills section is designed to help you settle quickly into your childcare course, and develop an understanding of how best to manage your learning, and integrate it with your personal life. Throughout your course you will be required to work independently on a variety of projects and assignments. The use of the various learning resources is covered here, as well as the various components of project planning.

Topic webs

This section of the book consists of 27 double page spreads representing the key components on the childcare curriculum. The left hand page of each spread introduces the topic, provides guidance on the resources available to study the area in greater detail, and lists postal and internet addresses of the various organisations who may be able to provide further information. It is a good idea to access the websites for information before telephoning or writing to any organisations as they are frequently very busy, and you will save them – and yourself – the time and expense of a postal enquiry.

The right hand page consists of a topic web which provides a pictorial outline of the relevant subject. The topic webs will give you an overview of the curriculum, and the basic terminology you will find useful in each area of study. You will note that many of the terms on each web are in bold, and it is these terms that you will find defined and explained in the next section – the childcare dictionary.

The childcare dictionary

The dictionary section provides the definition of those emboldened terms from the topic webs, and many, many more that you will encounter on your course. In all, approximately 1,000 terms are explained, and each term is fully cross referenced to other related words.

The authors are conscious that the choice of terms chosen for this type of dictionary must be subjective, and feel sure that others would have included different terminology on the one hand, whilst discarding others that we have submitted. We would be most grateful for any suggestions for additional, or replacement, terms, and ask that these be submitted through the publisher for consideration for any subsequent edition.

PART ONE: STUDY SKILLS

This section covers:

- Personal management
- Classroom learning
- Learning resources
- Project planning

The study skills section is designed to help you settle quickly into your childcare course, and develop an understanding of how best to manage your learning, and integrate it with your personal life.

Throughout your course work you will be required to work independently on a variety of projects and assignments, and in a variety of settings. As well as attending classroom sessions where groups of students will discuss and develop ideas with specialist lecturers, you will be expected to find and use a variety of sources of information and ideas. The use of the various learning resources is covered here, as well as the various components of project planning.

Knowing how to study effectively can make the difference between success and failure. This section, we hope, will help get you off to a good start.

Personal management

Before starting a course of study you will need to consider how to manage your personal and social life, so that you are able to meet the demands placed on you. Making plans to manage your more complicated life will enable you to succeed in gaining your qualification. It is important that you attempt to discover as much as possible about the course and its requirements, prior to making any commitment. It is a good idea to meet students who are still on the course so that you can ask questions about any elements that are worrying you.

Relationships

With family and friends

Many students have found that it is easier to be successful on an educational programme if they have the encouragement and support of partners, parents, children and friends. Before starting a course you will need to know the requirements of the course and discuss them fully with all concerned. This way, you will be sure of help when you most need it.

1

TO THINK ABOUT

Who will be most affected by your new commitment?
Who will offer most support?

Some students will enjoy their studies so much that other people in their lives may feel excluded and left behind. It takes a great deal of tact to resolve this predicament. There will be help available at most colleges, as tutors are familiar with this difficulty

With your college peer group

During the period of your course, you will be working closely with twenty or so people, engaging in interactive learning. You will all be expected to make positive contributions to discussion, and help maintain the security and confidence of the group. You may find yourself with people from different backgrounds, ages, different levels of maturity, and differing abilities. It may take you some time to settle in your group, but you will soon relax and enjoy the company of most of the people. Communicating with everyone in the group will broaden your ideas and attitudes.

As you will find in your training placement, you will be expected to display a professional attitude and enjoy the diversity of the group. The younger students will have plenty to learn from those with more experience of life, and the more mature students will appreciate listening to the views of the younger generation.

With tutors

Each group will have three or four subject teachers assigned to them, one of whom will act as personal tutor to the group. This tutor will be responsible for providing personal and group tutorial sessions. He or she may visit you in your training placement, discuss your progress and personal self-development, help you to sort out your problems, and write your reports.

All tutors will have different approaches and teaching styles and you may find that you are more comfortable with some tutors than with others. All tutors will have your interests at heart, and will be anxious for you to succeed.

During your induction, the college will make clear the roles and responsibilities of the tutors within the department. If you have a grievance of any sort, firstly take it up with the tutor involved and, if this does not prove to be successful, discuss the matter with your personal tutor.

Finances

Achieving any qualification will involve you in expense. Look at the chart on page 3 and work out your additional financial outlay.

There may be other expenses from time to time, such as money for entrance to exhibitions or museums, new social activities with the group and, of course, you will still have to maintain your living standards.

Fees for	
Tuition	
Registration: with college with validating body	
Exams	
Assessment	
Materials	
Costs	
Books	
Stationery	
Travel/fares	
Childcare	
Clothes: for placement for college	

Fees and costs

Many of you will be under the age of 19, and will not have to pay tuition fees, but will have to budget for the other costs. You may feel it is necessary to take a part-time job, or work during some of your holidays. Those of you over the age of 19 will find it increasingly difficult in the current financial climate to find a local authority prepared to give you a discretionary award, although some colleges will offer concessionary fees to some students. Some of you may have to give up a full- or part-time job, while others of you may lose your entitlement to state benefits. You will need to think very seriously about how you will meet the costs of the course and your living expenses. Many colleges have student advisors who will be able to help you and provide you with details of local and national charities that might be prepared to fund you, but applications must be well planned and on time in order to be successful.

Time management

The key to success lies in the way you manage your time.

The professional approach

Your time keeping will be a crucial factor in assessing your professional competence. It will be expected that you arrive punctually in college and in your placement. You will need to have planned your journey, and allowed plenty of time to ensure that you do not let anyone down by arriving late. Your attendance record will be monitored as no one will want to employ a person who is frequently absent or late, for whatever reason.

If being late or absent is unavoidable, you must make contact as soon as possible, explaining your predicament, and make sure that you keep in touch at regular intervals until the crisis has passed.

Organising your time when studying

This is a key factor in ensuring success. It will be expected that you will spend much of your personal time in:

- organising notes, portfolios and files
- further reading
- writing assignments
- planning and completing work undertaken in placement
- writing up your observations of children
- preparing individual and group presentations
- using the learning resource centre
- revising for tests
- keeping a diary.

If you are not in the habit of keeping a diary, you will now find it an essential tool to help you manage your time.

GOOD PRACTICE IN KEEPING A DIARY

1   Keep one diary only, with all your engagements in it.

2   Keep it with you all the time.

3   Fill in all long-term information and arrangements as soon as you have the diary, for example holiday and placement dates and times, and submission of assignment dates.

4   Fill in new arrangements as soon as you make them, for example dates of appointments and meetings.

5   Fill in information you may need when away from home, such as details of your next of kin, GP, bank, children's schools, your National Insurance number, placement telephone number and name of supervisor, and any other significant addresses and telephone numbers.

6   Keep a copy of your college timetable in the diary.

7   Keep the diary neat and up to date. You may decide to divide the day into three sections. Blank or cross out anything that has changed.

8   Use a thick elastic band around the front cover and used pages, so that the diary opens at the current week.

9   Paste an envelope in the back in which to keep tickets and appointment cards.

Look at the diary every day, and at the end of the day, to see what is planned for tomorrow, and to allow you time to prepare yourself.

GOOD PRACTICE IN MANAGING YOUR TIME

1   Obtain details of deadlines well in advance, and plan to finish your project ahead of time.
2   Keep up to date with all aspects of your work.
3   File your work on a daily basis.
4   Decide on the time of day that you are most alert and able to concentrate, and plan your study time to coincide with this.
5   Note in your diary dates of any tests or deadlines; avoid planning major social events at these times if possible.

Organising your social and leisure time

There will be less time for socialising once you have entered a course of study, so you will want to make the most of it. It is important that you have time for yourself, your family and friends to make sure that they do not feel excluded by your new life, and that your interests in leisure pursuits are sustained. Try to make time for regular exercise as this will help to offset stress. A life that is all work is a dull one to offer the children in your placement.

Resources and equipment

Essential equipment

- pens and pencils
- ruler
- rubber
- highlighter pens
- A4 paper, lined with punched holes
- A4 ring binders (at least 4, to start with)
- a strong bag or case to carry your work
- a diary
- a good general dictionary.

Suggestions for additional equipment

- scissors
- sticky tape
- glue or paste
- hole punch
- A4 plastic wallets
- a small notebook
- a stapler
- books.

The college will give you a list of the essential books that you will need to acquire to help you succeed on the course. It is a good idea to obtain these before the first day. Other books, perhaps on an optional list, you could order from libraries, or request them as presents from your family and friends. Bring and buy sales and charity shops are often a good source for cheap second hand books. If you own the books yourself, you will be able to highlight the passages of essential information. Having done this, it will be easier for you to find the relevant material when you come to write your assignments.

Childcare and educational theories are constantly changing and you will find it interesting to keep up with all the current issues by reading professional magazines, quality newspapers, watching television documentaries, and listening to discussions on the radio.

The home learning environment

Much of your study time will be away from college, and you will need to consider the following.

- Is there a room or a space where you can work without being interrupted?
- Is there a table or desk big enough for you to spread out your work undisturbed?
- Do you have a comfortable chair?
- Is your environment quiet, warm, well lit and well ventilated?
- Do you have shelving for your books and files?
- Do you have storage for your completed work?

If it is not ideal for you to study at home, for whatever reason, investigate the possibility of studying at a friend's house, or at your local library. Regular access to a computer would be helpful.

Stress management

As a student, you will often find yourself under considerable stress. The main causes may be some of the following.

- Conflicting demands on your time – juggling family commitments with assignment deadlines.
- Difficulty with the college work and meeting professional standards.
- Unclear about the expectations of tutors.
- Not feeling relaxed in the placement.
- Frequent absences from college, leading to lack of information and inability to complete assignments.
- Tensions in your relationships with your peer group, tutors or supervisors.
- Coming to terms with the student role.
- Coping with a reduction in your income.
- Coping with criticism and, perhaps, failure.
- Personal problems unrelated to the course.

Signs of stress

Your stress level may be indicated by tension headaches, variation in appetite, insomnia, tiredness, tearfulness, lack of concentration, inability to decide priorities and make decisions, and suppressed anger.

Managing stress

It is important to recognise and face up to the fact that you are stressed, and you need to attempt to identify the causes. Think about the following.

- Arrange to see your personal tutor to discuss your problems. He or she will assist you in devising an action plan.
- Arrange an appointment with your GP to discuss your symptoms and see what sources of help are available.
- Arrange an appointment with the student counsellor to consider a programme of counselling, to help you reflect and perhaps make changes in your lifestyle.
- Find out about assertiveness and relaxation techniques.
- Look again at how you are managing your time.
- Look at your diet and exercise regime.

It is perfectly normal to feel stress as a student. You are being constantly assessed and evaluated, both academically and in your professional development. The placement requires a strong commitment and it is very tiring working with children, particularly initially. As you progress on the course and increase your communication skills the stress should become more manageable.

Appeals and complaints

Grievances and complaints usually occur when there has been a breakdown in communication between the student and the tutors. This occurs rarely, but if it does your tutors will be as anxious as you to resolve it as quickly as possible. Colleges will have grievance procedures to follow, and are likely to bring them to your attention during the induction period. Representatives from the student union are available to help you put your case.

If you feel you have grounds for an appeal, in the event that you fail any part of the course, the validating body such as CACHE or BTEC will operate an appeals procedure. CACHE states that the appeals procedure must embody the principles of:

- natural justice
- fairness
- equity
- independence
- objectivity
- equal opportunities.

Your college tutors should acquaint you with the college and the validating body's appeals procedure when you first attend college.

Classroom learning

You know more than you think. You will already have achieved many things in your life, not necessarily all of them academic.

ACTIVITY

List your achievements and experiences to date.
What were the three easiest things you learnt to do? Why?
What were the three hardest things you learnt to do? Why?

To succeed on any course of study, you will need to understand the variety of techniques used in the classroom and the dynamics of different groups. A good tutor will use a number of different approaches in most lessons, and you will need to be adaptable and flexible so as to maximise your learning.

Taking dictation

If your tutor needs to convey to you some precise information, he or she might decide to dictate notes to you for a short period of time. This technique would not be used very often in most colleges. You will need to have pen and paper and to sit where you can hear clearly and see the board as the tutor may write certain words to ensure correct spelling. If you find it difficult to keep up with the pace, you should discuss it with the tutor.

Note-taking

During many classes and lectures, your tutor will be addressing the whole class, introducing topics, discussing new theories and examining controversial arguments and you will be expected to take notes of the most important points. Your tutor will probably adopt one of two modes of delivery. He or she might explain what has to be covered in a particular topic, deliver the lecture, and then confirm what has been covered in the lesson. On the other hand, your tutor might adopt an argumentative approach by introducing an issue and then stating arguments for and arguments against, finally summarising points for and against and attempting to come to some conclusion. To take notes well you should do the following.

- Be on time.
- Have pens, paper and highlighters to hand.
- Sit where you can see and hear.
- Listen actively, not allowing yourself to be distracted.
- Be active, ask questions.
- Only write down important points, use your own shorthand.
- Make a note of any important questions (and answers) asked at the end of the lecture.
- Always go over the notes the same day, so that you can correct, revise, add or delete information.
- Date and file your notes.

Discussion in class

Sometimes your tutor will introduce a topic and then expect the group to spend some time contributing their own relevant ideas and experiences. This can be one of the best ways of understanding and learning the core elements of the course.

It is not always easy at first to have the confidence to speak within the group setting. You might be afraid that your ideas are not valid, and that the rest of the group might reject or make fun of your remarks. To benefit from group discussion you should do the following.

- Listen to other people respectfully and do not interrupt.
- Have pen and paper to jot down ideas as they occur to you.
- Indicate to the tutor that you wish to speak.
- Make sure your contribution is relevant to the discussion.
- Speak slowly and clearly.
- Try to avoid anecdotal evidence, particularly if it is going to cause you stress.
- Remember that nearly everybody feels nervous at first when contributing to a classroom discussion. It becomes easier with practice.

Seminars/presentations

You may be asked, during the course, to present a seminar paper, or make a presentation to the group, either on your own or with two or three other students. You will need to be clear about the purpose of the presentation, what you wish to communicate and how you are going to present the information. Remember to speak clearly, audibly and slowly enough so that the group has time to take in what you are saying. Face the group at all times, even if you are using visual aids. Remember to:

- be yourself, and find your own style
- be positive
- accept that you will be nervous beforehand and try some relaxation techniques
- concentrate on the task, remembering what you are trying to communicate
- monitor your vocal expression, thinking about volume, pitch and pace
- articulate your words more clearly for a larger audience
- avoid too many statistics. If necessary, put them in a handout and ask the tutor to photocopy it for you
- check any visual aids such as overhead projectors beforehand
- never apologise for your presentation
- try to rehearse with friends before the actual presentation.

Role play

While on your course, you may be asked to take on the role of another person, so that you can begin to experience the feelings and emotions that someone might feel in a certain situation. This is unlikely to occur until the group has settled and the tutor has a good understanding of the group dynamic.

Your tutor will brief you very clearly as to what is expected of you. Usually, role play will be between two people, with a third one observing what is happening. The observer will then report back to the other two. On occasion, for example if you were role playing the child protection conference, a larger group would be involved, and the rest of the class would observe. It is always important to have feedback, and for the participants to have the opportunity to state how they felt. Taking on the role of others improves your ability to see other people's points of view. This ability is called 'empathy' and is different from feeling sympathetic, as it allows you to enter into the emotions of another person. To speculate on the emotions of others and to apply them to oneself is an integral part of professional development.

Brainstorming

Brainstorming is the term used where a number of people are expected to contribute ideas to a particular topic in a spontaneous and fast fashion. This will help enrich a subject with creative, lateral and original thinking. All ideas are accepted, however wild or extravagant they may seem at first.

Someone is generally elected (the scribe) to record the ideas on a large sheet of paper, or on a board, while another person acts as chairperson so as to keep some order in the proceedings. Everyone in the group is expected to participate in a positive fashion. The chairperson should prevent any negative attitudes, as this will inhibit creativity. The group may decide to set a time limit. The scribe will read back the list to the group on request and at the end of the initial session.

The group will then classify the entire list, combining and improving ideas. They may discover gaps in the topic and some areas may have been over subscribed. The tutor may intervene and suggest unexplored concepts. A general discussion will follow and the ideas will be evaluated in a positive way. The value of brainstorming is that:

- it helps you to think about what you already know about a particular topic before taking on fresh ideas
- it allows the whole class to contribute without inhibition
- it allows free expression and spontaneity
- negativity is ruled out
- some students explore thoughts and ideas that they would not do on their own
- classifying and evaluating ideas is a useful exercise in organising one's own work.
- working as a group on a topic demonstrates the value of teamwork.

Using worksheets with videos

As a student on a childcare course, you will need knowledge and understanding of many different children, from different backgrounds, with different needs, of different ages and in different settings. To supplement your practical training, your tutor may wish you to watch a number of videos. This is not a passive exercise, and you will be expected to take notes on what you are watching, sometimes complete worksheets and join in discussion in a critical fashion. Always note the title, date and publisher of the video, as you may wish to include it in a bibliography.

When you first start to observe children, your tutor may ask the group to watch a short extract from a video, record their observations, and report to the group what they have observed, noting the range of different perceptions.

You should document and file your video notes with your class notes.

To help you become more adept at close observation of video recordings, you might find it useful to watch a relevant television documentary at home and take notes.

Functioning in different types of groups

Small groups

From time to time, your tutor may ask you to work in small groups of four or five to complete a particular task. You will be given pens and flip chart paper, or acetate and acetate pens, and one of you will record the ideas and findings of your group. Towards the end of the session, one of you will report back to the larger group. You will need to make your own notes of the whole session, so that you can document and file the work for future use.

Your class group

When starting the course, you will be placed in a group of approximately twenty people. This is the size of group for most of your teaching sessions. As you spend time together, you will become familiar with the group dynamics and behaviour. You will no doubt make some firm friendships.

Large lecture groups

Cuts in further education budgets and the reduction of course hours have resulted in groups of forty or more students attending some lectures for part of the curriculum delivery. So as to get the most from these sessions you will need to behave in a more formal manner. You must be punctual, sitting down as quickly as possible, and being as quiet as you can. There is much less interaction between the tutor and individual members of the group. You will be expected to take notes and file them as described at the beginning of this section. There may be some time towards the end of the session to ask questions, but if you run out of time or you are too diffident to speak in such a large group, make sure you record your queries, so that you can raise the issue in a general class session.

Whatever the size of the group, you will be required to make a positive contribution. The dynamics in the group will vary, with some people speaking more than others, but everyone is expected to take part in some way.

Learning resources

The learning resource centre

Learning resource centres have evolved from traditional libraries which just carried books, to provide opportunities for students to study and research using all the current technology. In any learning resource centre you will find sections for:

- fiction books
- non-fiction books
- reference books
- journals and newspapers
- new additions to stock
- storage of information files, including press cuttings and handouts
- classifying the stock, such as catalogues and indices
- audio and visual material, such as audio books and videos
- computers and CD-Roms.

At the start of your course you will be shown how to use the learning resource centre. You will be shown how to use the Dewey Decimal System, which classifies the books and helps you to find them on the shelves. You will be given instruction in the catalogue system, which will cross-reference authors, titles and subjects. The catalogue system might use index cards but the information will more likely be held on computers.

You will need to become familiar with the facilities and be prepared to ask questions and employ the skills of the professional staff if there is any area which is new to you. You will probably be spending a fair proportion of your time studying on your own, researching and preparing material for assignments.

The learning resource centre should be a quiet place of study, and it is important that you respect this, and use other more appropriate areas of the college in which to socialise.

Literature searches

You may have access to databases through the learning resource centre that catalogues books and articles held there. A profile of relevant articles may be identified in response to key terms, and this may provide a quick way to find pertinent information. Your learning resource centre advisor can tell you which databases are available and how to use them.

Using information technology

Most of you will be familiar with computers, either from home or from school. You may find that information technology 'Key Skills' is incorporated into your course and you will quickly appreciate the value of this skill in writing assignments and observations and being able to help the children in your placements. If you do not have access to a PC at home, you will be able to book sessions in the learning resource centre.

Access to the internet, either at college or at home, will help you with your research enabling you to access a wide range of up-to-date information. It will often give you a synopsis of books that you might want to read. Organisations such as the NSPCC and Kidscape will have web sites, and this is helpful in providing information quickly.

Check what CD-Roms are available as these can be invaluable in your understanding of certain topics.

Booklists

At the start of any course you may be given a list of essential books that you will need to obtain to successfully complete your area of study. It is sensible to try to buy these as there will be competing demands on the library stock, and they are probably on the list because you will need to refer to them throughout the course, at college and at home. Other books, on optional booklists relating to specific modules, may be ordered from your local library.

Handouts

Frequently your tutors will distribute handouts about various areas of the work and will either read them through in class with you, or expect you to study them on your own. This saves time in dictating important material. You can highlight any particular points that you or your tutor feel to be of vital interest, and this will help you later on when you might be writing an assignment. All handouts should be dated and filed with your course material.

Using books for research

As you know, all text books have a table of contents indicating the sequence of chapters and lists of charts and illustrations, and some will also have appendices, footnotes, bibliographies and an index. When selecting a book look at the following.

- The introduction or preface. These may give you some idea what the book is about and at which level it is aimed.
- The contents or chapter headings. This will indicate the main topics or areas covered.
- The date of publication, which will tell you how up to date the work is.
- The summary or conclusions, which may give you some overview of the book.
- The index. If your topic is not mentioned in the contents, you may find it here.
- The bibliography. Some books will suggest further reading, as well as resources, references or useful addresses.
- The charts, diagrams, graphs and illustrations which may be of help in your project.

You may not be able to find all that you require on a particular topic in your college learning resource centre. Enrol in your local library where you will be able to order books and other resources for a small payment. Consider buying books in partnership with other members of your group and borrowing from people who have completed your course.

Other resources

Museums and exhibitions around the country offer resources and opportunities for extending your understanding and knowledge. Find out what is available in your local area and seize the opportunity to subscribe to any free mailing list. Your tutor will probably arrange some group visits and you will find that your learning will be greatly enriched.

Your placement will have some days set aside for training (INSET days). You will find these extremely valuable. If the dates clash with a college day, your tutor will probably give you permission to attend and may wish you to feed the information back to the group at a later date.

The magazine *Nursery World* organises exhibitions of resources, books and equipment, for under-eights in London and in other parts of the country. These exhibitions are particularly valuable as they keep you up to date, offer programmes of seminars on current issues, and allow you to meet a number of different people involved in working with young children.

Project planning

You will be assessed on your course by a series of assignments that you will be expected to complete by a given date. The assignments may take the form of essays, presentations or projects. These tasks require careful long-term planning, research and recording.

Filing work

One way of making sure that your course of study is a success is to have easy access to your material. All those notes that you so carefully wrote down, all those hand-outs given to you in class and those activities that you have planned and carried out in your placement – all this needs to be carefully sorted and filed. All written work that you complete needs to be dated, titled and carry your name.

There are several methods of filing your course work. Most students prefer a different file for each subject (education, health, social studies and so on). Within each subject you may choose one or both of the following methods.

- Date order (chronological): each piece of work is added to the file in date order, with the date in the top right hand corner of the page.
- Topic headings: most subjects are broken down into topics. For example, in your education file, you might put pre-school provision and the National Curriculum. In your health file, you might put nutrition and physical growth and development. In your social studies file, you might put the Children Act, 1989, and notes on the family. This is a convenient method of filing but be careful not to view each topic in isolation.

Some students might find it useful to keep a list of contents at the front of the file for quick access. The use of dividers in different colours, with the name of each topic clearly depicted is another useful way of finding what you need quickly.

Portfolios

The word 'portfolio' is used to describe the folder that contains evidence demonstrating your ability to work competently and skilfully with young children. Your tutor will indicate as you commence the course how you should compile your portfolios. The Certificate in Childcare and Education requires certain information to be included in your portfolio. If you are studying the Diploma in Nursery Nursing, Module A and Module B require separate portfolios with specific information. It is important to listen to your tutor, question anything you do not understand, and follow instructions carefully when compiling portfolios.

Assignments

Essays

An essay is a piece of writing on a specific subject. It may be long or short, it may be written at home or under a time constraint. If you are writing the essay at home, you will be asked to limit it to a certain number of words.

When writing an essay on any subject, you need to be clear that you are:

- responding clearly to the instructions in the essay title

- drawing on the relevant parts of the course
- showing a good understanding of the subject
- presenting a coherent argument
- using an objective style
- introducing appropriate evidence to support your argument
- attempting to present your work in a legible, easy to read style, with few spelling or grammatical errors.

It is helpful to follow the general essay plan shown on page 16.

Presentations

Presentations include seminars, interviews and role plays which have been prepared to perform in front of your group and tutors. They will show an understanding of work that you have done in some topic area. They need to be carefully planned and researched. This will increase your confidence in presenting work to a group. You may be asked to present a transcript of your presentation.

Projects

A project is usually a longer piece of work than an essay, and requires research and planning. Colleges should carry up to date information and resources within the learning resource centre. If the assignment is one that is being given to all students across the country, organisations will find it difficult to cope with thousands of requests for information. You might find it more profitable and a great deal faster to access the internet for the information you require.

Having been set an assignment clarify:

- what you are required to do
- what information you need to complete the assignment
- where you will find this information
- the date of submission of the work.

If the assignment requires you to undertake a piece of work or research in your placement, you should discuss it with your supervisor as soon as possible, and arrange a time and date to complete the work. Try to have a clear idea of how long the project will take, allowing time to proofread the first draft and make any necessary amendments before submitting the finished assignment. Your work needs to be presented as attractively as possible, preferably typed or word-processed, using double spacing on A4 paper, and securely bound.

Referencing

You will obviously need to use and refer to other people's work when writing any type of assignment. You must, however, be very careful to avoid the temptation to plagiarise. This means copying chunks of text and using it as your own work, without adequate referencing or any acknowledgement.

It is important that you use references within your text. The Harvard System is shown in Appendix C, as circulated by CACHE. All assignments that you write will require a bibliography. This will include all books, videos and articles that you have quoted, listed in alphabetical order. It may also include books that you have used for background reading.

GENERAL ESSAY PLAN

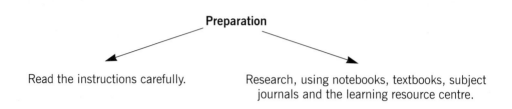

Preparation

Read the instructions carefully.

Research, using notebooks, textbooks, subject journals and the learning resource centre.

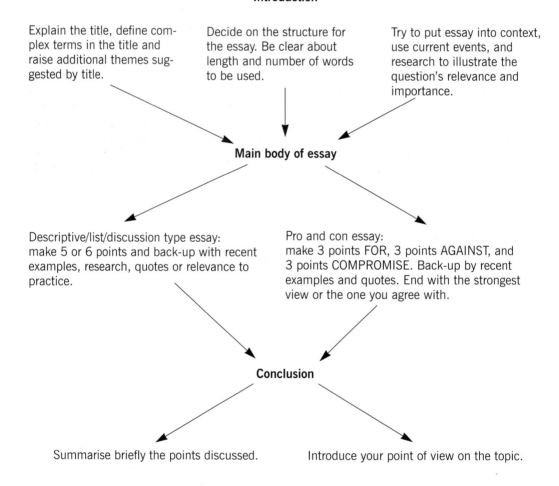

Introduction

Explain the title, define complex terms in the title and raise additional themes suggested by title.

Decide on the structure for the essay. Be clear about length and number of words to be used.

Try to put essay into context, use current events, and research to illustrate the question's relevance and importance.

Main body of essay

Descriptive/list/discussion type essay: make 5 or 6 points and back-up with recent examples, research, quotes or relevance to practice.

Pro and con essay: make 3 points FOR, 3 points AGAINST, and 3 points COMPROMISE. Back-up by recent examples and quotes. End with the strongest view or the one you agree with.

Conclusion

Summarise briefly the points discussed.

Introduce your point of view on the topic.

NB Remember to include your references and bibliography.

Controlled assignments

During the course you will be given dates when you will be asked to write controlled assignments relating to certain modules. You will be given the titles about two weeks before these dates. You will have this time to prepare and research the subject thoroughly, and will then write the essay under timed examination conditions in college.

Multiple choice questions (MCQs)

These are questions posed to students where one of four presented answers is the correct one. You will indicate the one you think is correct. Any MCQ paper will consist of a specific number of questions and you will be given a period of time to complete the paper. Generally questions will test your knowledge or your practice. Your tutor will prepare you for this test, and will indicate how you are to record your response. If you do not know the answer to any question immediately, it is good sense to leave it, answer all the ones you do know, and in the time left, tackle the ones you are not sure about. Most tutors will ensure that you have plenty of practice with mock papers to develop and improve your technique.

Assessment procedures

As a childcare student, you will be assessed during and at the end of the course, in your academic achievements and progress, in your professional development and competence and in your practical work. It is necessary that you understand that your assessment starts from the first day of the course, and you need to be clear about the expectations of your tutors, the college and the validating body. Many validating bodies issue an overview of their requirements and procedures and it is in your interest to obtain a copy of this document.

Additional resources

Northedge, A., *The Good Study Guide*, Open University, 1990

PART TWO: TOPIC WEBS

This section contains topic information and webs on the following areas.

1 The needs of children	14 Play
2 The newborn	15 Early years education
3 Working with babies	16 Activities with children
4 Emotional development	17 Partnership with parents
5 Language development	18 Safety
6 Social development	19 Child protection
7 Cognitive development	20 Food and nutrition
8 Physical development and growth	21 Prevention of infection
	22 The sick child
9 Challenging behaviour	23 Children and society
10 Personal development	24 Children with disabilities
11 Equal opportunities	25 Employment
12 Observations	26 Maintaining good health in children
13 Pre-school provision	27 Playwork

The aim of this section is to give you as much guidance as possible in the planning of project and assignment work and consists of 27 double page spreads representing the key components of the childcare curriculum.

The left hand page of each spread introduces the topic, provides guidance on the resources available to study the area in greater detail, and lists postal and internet addresses of the various organisations that may be able to provide further information. It is a good idea to access the websites for information before telephoning or writing to any organisations as they are frequently very busy, and you will save them – and yourself – the time and expense of a postal enquiry.

The right hand page consists of a topic web which provides a pictorial outline of the relevant subject. The topic webs will give you an overview of the curriculum, and the basic terminology you will find useful in each area of study. You will note that many of the terms on each web are in bold, and it is these terms that you will find defined and explained in the next section – the childcare dictionary.

1 The needs of children

When working with children, it is important to understand that there is a variety of needs that have to be met before children are able to grow and develop satisfactorily and achieve their full potential. It is necessary to maintain a balance and adopt a holistic approach in caring for children.

Children belong to many different and diverse groups, with different values, religions, and approaches to child-rearing. However, all children need love and security, stimulation and education, routine physical care and the right to protection.

Frequent monitoring and observation of children will help you to focus on these basic needs. If you should identify any child whose needs are not being met in any area, you will be able to take appropriate action.

Resources

Beaver, M. et al, *The Development of Babies and Young Children: 0–7*, Stanley Thornes, 1994
   Babies and Young Children: Work and Care (2nd edn), Stanley Thornes, 1999
Bee, H., *The Developing Child* (8th edn), Addison-Wesley, 1997
   The Growing Child, HarperCollins, 1995
Bruce, T., *Tuning in to Children*, BBC Education, 1996
Fisher, J., *Starting from the Child*, Open University, 1996
Flanagan, Cara, *Applying Psychology to Early Child Development*, Hodder & Stoughton, 1996
Illingworth, R. and Illingworth, C., *Babies and Young Children* (7th edn), Churchill Livingstone, 1984
Kellmer Pringle, Mia, *The Needs of Children* (3rd edn), Routledge, 1986
Leach, P., *Children First*, Michael Joseph, 1994
   Baby and Child, Penguin, 1988
Lynch, E. and Hanson, M., *Developing Cross Cultural Competence*, Paul M. Brookes Pub. Co, 1992
McIlveen, R. and Gross, R., *Developmental Psychology*, Hodder & Stoughton, 1997
Morgan, S. and Righton, P., *Child Care: Concerns and Conflicts*, Hodder & Stoughton with Open University, 1989
O'Hagan, M. and Smith, M., *Special Issues in Childcare*, Baillière Tindall, 1993
Stoppard, M., *Complete Baby and Child Care*, Dorling Kindersley, 1995

Addresses

The Children's Society, Edward Rudolph House, Marjery Street, London WC1. Telephone: 0171 837 4299. Website: http://www.the-childrens-society.org.UK
The National Children's Bureau, 8 Wakely Street, London EC1V 7QE. Telephone: 0171 843 6000. Website: www.ncb.org.UK
The National Early Years Network, 77 Holloway Road, Islington, London N7 8JZ. Telephone: 0171 607 9573. Website: www.ncb.org.UK
National Children's Home Action for Children. Website: www.nchafc.org.UK

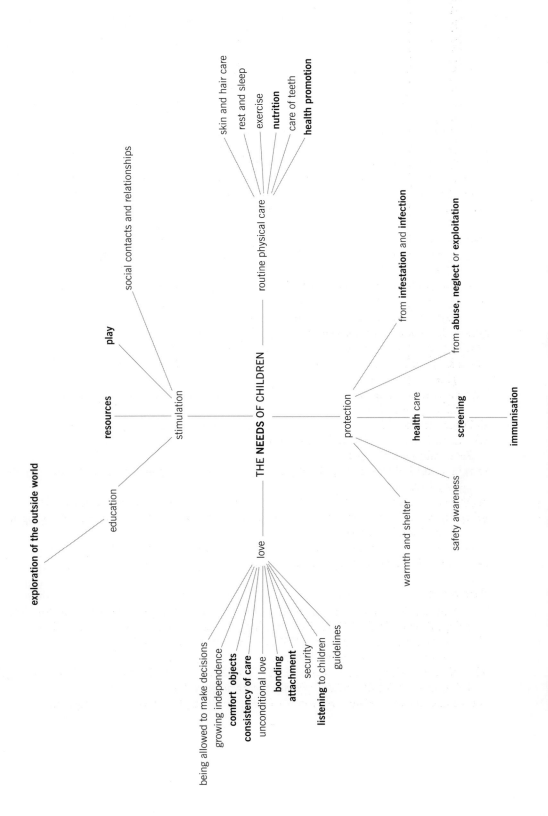

skin and hair care

rest and sleep

exercise

nutrition

care of teeth

health promotion

social contacts and relationships

routine physical care

from **infestation** and **infection**

from **abuse, neglect** or **exploitation**

play

exploration of the outside world

resources

stimulation

THE NEEDS OF CHILDREN

protection

health care

screening

immunisation

education

love

warmth and shelter

safety awareness

being allowed to make decisions

growing independence

comfort objects

consistency of care

unconditional love

bonding

attachment

security

listening to children

guidelines

2 The newborn

Unlike the growing area of working with babies, there are few job opportunities working with the neonate, which describes the first four weeks of life. It is important to understand pre-conceptual and antenatal care, as you may find yourself supporting parents who are expecting new additions to the family.

As a childcare practitioner, you may work with newborn babies in obstetric units or, after gaining some experience, in the home setting as a maternity nurse. In the hospital you may be asked to carry out some procedures for which you have not been trained, such as the Guthrie test or tube feeding the baby. You must discuss this with your line manager and ensure you receive adequate training in all unfamiliar procedures. Check your insurance cover.

The mother and, indeed, all the family, need time to bond successfully with the newborn baby, and your awareness of this will prevent you from becoming over-involved. Promoting this attachment in a sensitive way will be one of your priorities. If this is the first child in the family, the mother may need help and advice about routine physical care, and how to fulfil the emotional needs of her baby.

Resources
Johnston, P., *The Newborn Child* (8th edn), Churchill Livingstone, 1998
Leach, P., *Babyhood*, Penguin, 1991
Nilsson, L., *A Child is Born*, Doubleday, 1994
Robertson, J. and Robertson, J., *A Baby in the Family*, Harmondsworth, Penguin, 1982
Williams, F., *Babycare for Beginners*, HarperCollins, 1996

Addresses
Association for Post Natal Illness, 25 Jerdan Place, London SW6 1BE. Telephone: 0171 386 0868
Birth Defects Foundation, Chelsea House, Westgate, London LO5 1DN. Telephone: 0181 862 0198
Cry-sis, BM Crysis, London WC1N 3XX. Telephone: 0171 404 5011
National Childbirth Trust (NCT), Alexandra House, Oldham Terrace, London W3 6NH. Telephone: 0181 992 8637
Stillbirth and Neonatal Death Society (SANDS) 28 Portland Place, London W1N 4 DE. Telephone: 0171 436 7940. Website: http://members.aul,co,\babyloss\sands.htm
Twins and Multiple Births Association, PO Box 30, Little Sutton, South Wirrall L66 1TH. Telephone: 0151 348 0020. Website: http://www.surreyweb.org.UK/TAMBA

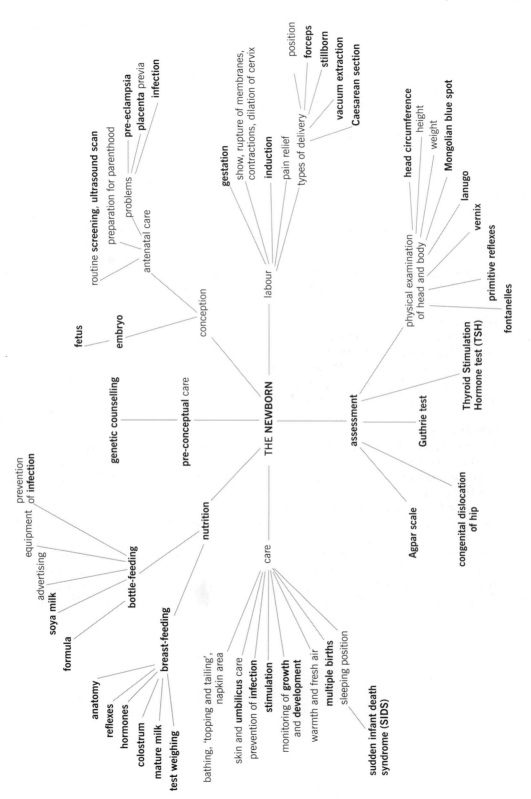

THE NEWBORN

conception

genetic counselling

pre-conceptual care

fetus

embryo

antenatal care

routine **screening, ultrasound scan**

preparation for parenthood

problems

pre-eclampsia

placenta previa

infection

labour

gestation

show, rupture of membranes, contractions, dilation of cervix

induction

pain relief

types of delivery

position

forceps

stillborn

vacuum extraction

Caesarean section

assessment

physical examination of head and body

head circumference

height

weight

Mongolian blue spot

lanugo

vernix

primitive reflexes

fontanelles

Thyroid Stimulation Hormone test (TSH)

Guthrie test

Agpar scale

congenital dislocation of hip

nutrition

bottle-feeding

prevention of **infection**

equipment

advertising

soya milk

formula

breast-feeding

anatomy

reflexes

hormones

colostrum

mature milk

test weighing

care

bathing, 'topping and tailing', napkin area

skin and **umbilicus** care

prevention of **infection**

stimulation

monitoring of **growth** and **development**

warmth and fresh air

multiple births

sleeping position

sudden infant death syndrome (SIDS)

3 Working with babies

Changing lifestyles have resulted in more babies receiving routine care from people other than their mothers. Some babies remain in their own home with nannies while others are taken to child-minders. An increasing number will go into group care settings. Babies need very different routine care than older children, and consistent and familiar care is particularly important. You will realise that babies need a great deal of physical care, but you must not neglect their cognitive, emotional and social development

Resources
Bremner, J., *Infancy* (2nd edn), Blackwell, 1994
Bowlby, J., *Child Care and the Growth of Love*, Pelican, 1953
Cowley, L., *Young Children in Group Daycare* (2nd edn), NCB, 1994
Dare, A., and O'Donovan, M., *Working with Babies* (2nd edn), Stanley Thornes, 1998
Goldschmied, E., 'Play and learning in the first year of life' in Williams, V. (Ed.), *Babies in Daycare*, Daycare Trust, 1989
Goldschmied, E., and Jackson, S., *People Under Three*, Routledge, 1994
Miller, L., Rustin, M. and M., and Shuttleworth, J. (Eds), *Closely Observed Infants*, Duckworth, 1989
PLA, *Play and Learning for Under Threes*, PLA Promotion, 45–49 Union Road, Croydon, CR0 2XU
Sheridan, M., *From Birth to Five Years* (revised and updated by Frost, M. and Sharma, A.), Routledge, 1997
Talbot, J. (Ed.), *Infant Feeding: the First Year*, Profile Productions, 1989
Valman, H.B., *The First Year of Life* (4th edn), BMJ Publishing Group, 1995
Wolfson, R., *The professional nanny guide*, Nursery World Publications, 1997

Training videos
Goldschmied, E., *Infants at Work*, NCB, 1986
Goldschmied, E. and Hughes, A., *Heuristic Play with Objects*, NCB, 1992

Addresses
Foundation for the Study of Infant Deaths, 15 Belgrave Square, London SW1X 8PS. Telephone: 0171 235 0965/1721. Website: www.vois.org.UK/FSID
Multiple Birth Foundation, Queen Charlotte's and Chelsea Hospital, Goldhawk Road, London W6 0XG. Telephone: 0181 748 4666.

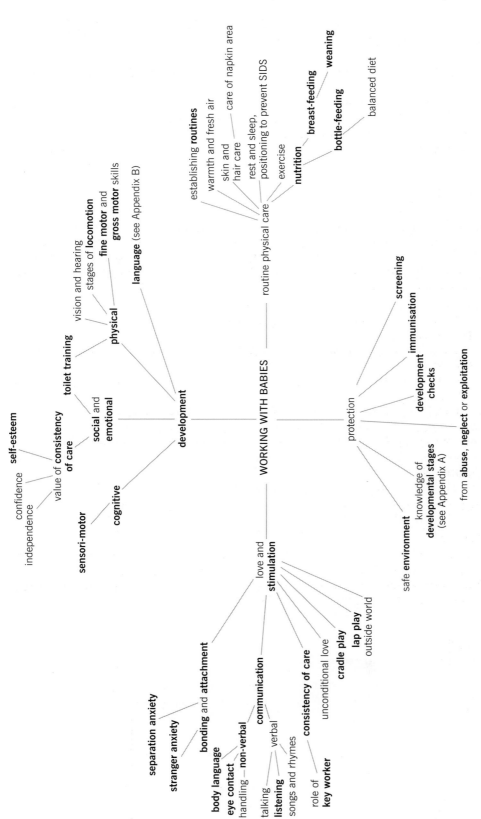

WORKING WITH BABIES

development

routine physical care

protection

development

physical

social and emotional

cognitive

sensori-motor

physical

vision and hearing

stages of **locomotion**

fine motor and **gross motor** skills

language (see Appendix B)

toilet training

value of **consistency of care**

self-esteem

confidence

independence

routine physical care

establishing **routines**

warmth and fresh air

skin and hair care

care of napkin area

rest and sleep, positioning to prevent SIDS

exercise

nutrition

breast-feeding

bottle-feeding

weaning

balanced diet

protection

screening

immunisation

development checks

knowledge of **developmental stages** (see Appendix A)

from **abuse**, **neglect** or **exploitation**

safe **environment**

love and **stimulation**

separation anxiety

stranger anxiety

bonding and **attachment**

body language

eye contact

handling — **non-verbal**

communication

talking — verbal

listening

songs and rhymes

role of **key worker**

consistency of care

unconditional love

cradle play

lap play

outside world

4 Emotional development

During your career as a childcare practitioner, you will become aware of the importance of building relationships with children, helping them to develop emotional strengths, and enabling them to reach adulthood confident in themselves and valuing their achievements.

From the moment of birth, the baby begins the process of attachment, bonding with the mother in the same way as the mother bonds with the baby. This love and mutual trust is the basis of emotional development, allowing the child to continue to make loving and trusting relationships with other members of the family and later with the outside world.

There will be times in the lives of the children in your care when you will need to be particularly sensitive. Settling a child successfully into a new situation often needs careful handling. The birth of a new baby may lead to feelings of jealousy and rejection. Problems within the child's family, such as divorce, unemployment, death or addiction may distress the child and halt emotional development, causing the child to regress.

Understanding the stages of emotional development is a critical factor in ensuring good practice.

Resources
Axline, V., *Dibs, In Search of Self*, Penguin, 1966
Bowlby, J., *Child Care and the Growth of Love* (2nd edn), Penguin, 1965
Flanagan, C., *Applying Psychology to Early Child Development*, Hodder & Stoughton, 1996
Goldschmied, E., *People Under Three*, Routledge, 1994
Hartley-Brewer, F., *Positive Parenting: Raising Children with Self-Esteem*, Vermilion, 1998
Pearce, J., *Worries and Fears*, Thorsons, 1989
Roberts, R., *Self-esteem and Successful Early Learning*, Hodder & Stoughton, 1995
Robertson, J. and Robertson, J., *Separation and the Very Young*, Free Association Books, 1989
Rutter, M., *Helping Troubled Children*, Penguin, 1975
    Maternal Deprivation Reassessed (2nd edn), Penguin, 1981
Wadsworth, B.J., *Piaget's Theory of Cognitive and Affective Development*, Longman, 1996
Winnicott, D., *The Child, the Family and the Outside World*, Penguin, 1964
Wolfson, R., *Sibling Rivalry*, Thorsons, 1995

Videos
Looking at Children's Brief Separations, series of 5 videos produced by the Robertsons. Concord Video and Film Council Ltd. Telephone: 01473 726 012

Theorists
John Bowlby, **Sigmund Freud**, **Carl Jung**

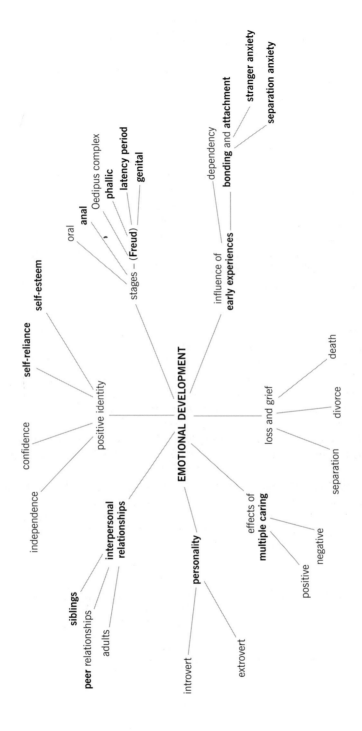

EMOTIONAL DEVELOPMENT

stages – (**Freud**)
oral
anal
Oedipus complex
phallic
latency period
genital

influence of **early experiences**
dependency
bonding and **attachment**
stranger anxiety
separation anxiety

positive identity
self-esteem
self-reliance
confidence
independence

interpersonal relationships
siblings
peer relationships
adults

personality
introvert
extrovert

effects of **multiple caring**
positive
negative

loss and grief
death
divorce
separation

5 Language development

Human beings are the only organisms that can converse fluently with each other and can read and write. The ability to communicate well is a key factor in happiness and achievement. The discovery of feral children has shown us that practice and exposure to language is essential from birth, and that without language it is not possible to grow and develop satisfactorily.

In all countries and cultures language development follows the same sequence (see Appendix B). A good knowledge of language development will help you to detect a child whose language is immature or delayed, and you will know how to help a child yourself and when to make an appropriate referral.

Children whose heritage language is not English have the enormous advantage of growing up speaking two languages fluently. On first entry to nursery or school they may need some support and additional help. Be careful not to assume that delay in acquiring English indicates that there is a delay in other areas of development. Access to books in their heritage language allows parents to read with the children. Fluency in the heritage language will enable them to become fluent in English later on.

Resources
Arnberg, L., *Raising Children Bilingually*, Multilingual Matters, 1987
Browne, A., *Helping Children to Write*, Paul Chapman, 1993
   Developing Language and Literacy, 3–8 years, Paul Chapman, 1996
Gravelle, M., *Supporting Bilingual Learning in Schools*, Trentham Books, 1997
Lock, A. and Fisher, E. (Eds), *Language Development*, OUP, 1984
Petrie, P., *Communicating with Children and Adults* (2nd edn), Arnold, 1997
Whitehead, M., *Language and Literacy in the Early Years*, Paul Chapman, 1990
   The Development of Language and Literacy, Hodder & Stoughton, 1996

CD Rom
'Sign Now' (teaches how to use British Sign Language) from Micro Books, 42 Beverley Road, Sunbury, Middlesex TW16 6TN. Telephone: 01932 882282

Addresses
National Deaf Children's Society, 15 Dufferin Street, London EC1Y 0PD. Telephone: 0171 250 0123
Royal College of Speech and Language Therapists, 7 Bath Place, Rivington Street, London EC2A 3DR. Telephone: 0171 613 3855. Website: http://www.rcslt.org.

Theorists
Noam Chomsky, Jean Piaget, Lev Vygotsky

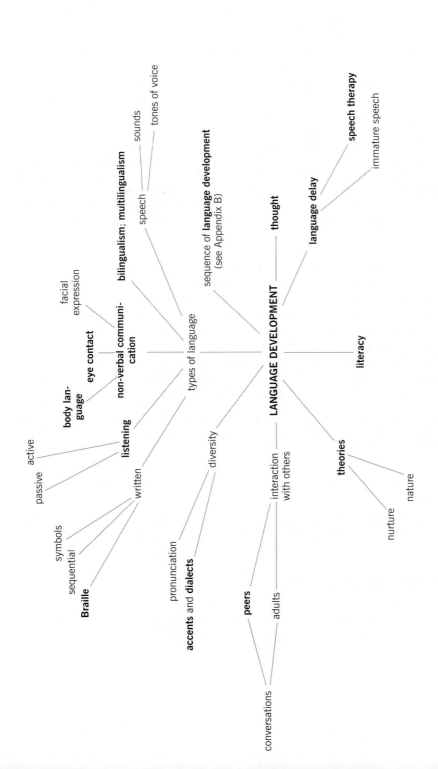

6 Social development

A human being is born without any social skills, and becoming a social being is learnt initially in the family, and then in the wider environment. Feral children who are brought up by animals or those locked away with no human contact, not only do not develop socially but also do not develop physical skills, such as walking and do not have any recognisable language. The existence of these children indicates clearly that all children need human contact to develop normally so that they can take their place in society.

Social development takes place alongside emotional development, and the importance of the environment cannot be over-emphasised. You will need to have a clear understanding of the stages and sequences of the child's developing relationships within society, the process of socialisation and the development of the child's social skills.

In our multicultural society, there are many different cultures with different beliefs and values. Knowledge of these cultures will help you to appreciate the richness of the society and the difficulties sometimes encountered by children who are coping with different value systems and customs at a very young age.

Resources

Barnes, P., (Ed.) *Personal, Social and Emotional Development of Children*, Blackwell, 1995
Dunn, J., *The Beginnings of Social Understanding*, Blackwell, 1988
    Young Children's Close Relationships, Sage, 1993
Goldschmied, E. and Selleck, D., *Communication between Babies in their First Year*, NCB 1996 (a video is included with this training book)
Gross, R., *Psychology* (3rd edn), Hodder & Stoughton, 1997
Oates, J., *The Foundations of Child Development*, OUP, 1994
Wolfson, R., *From Birth to Starting School*, Nursery World Publications, 1997

Theorist
Erik Erikson

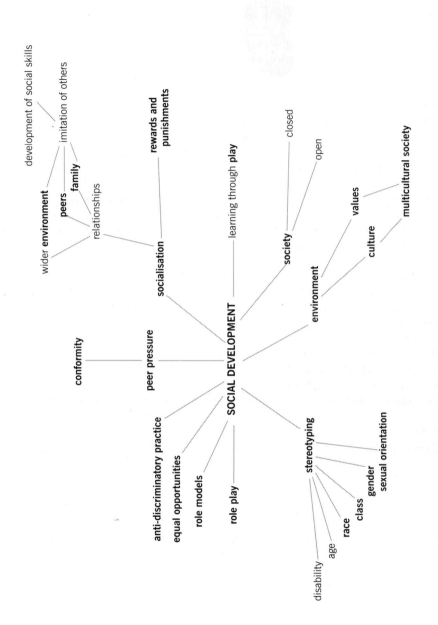

development of social skills

imitation of others

rewards and punishments

family

peers

wider environment

relationships

closed

open

society

learning through play

values

socialisation

culture

environment

multicultural society

conformity

peer pressure

SOCIAL DEVELOPMENT

anti-discriminatory practice

equal opportunities

role models

role play

stereotyping

disability

age

race

class

gender

sexual orientation

7 Cognitive development

Cognitive development, sometimes described as intellectual development, shows the way in which we learn to think. There are many theories as to how this takes place, but most would agree that the learning happens in stages and is sequential.

Some theorists believe that most cognitive ability is inherited, whereas others think that the influence of the environment is paramount. Piaget, the most influential of the theorists, argues that it is both.

You will need to understand age-appropriate activities so as to promote, encourage and extend children's learning and imagination. You will need to be conversant with the development of language (Appendix B: Sequence of language development), and be aware how this links with cognitive development.

Resources

Blenkin, G. and Kelly, A., (Eds), *Early Childhood Education* (2nd edn), Paul Chapman, 1996

Deakin, M., *Children on the Hill*, Quartet Books, 1973

de Bono, E., *Teach Your Child How to Think*, Viking (Penguin), 1992

Donaldson, M., *Children's Minds*, Fontana, 1978

Grieve, R. and Hughes, M. (Eds), *Understanding Children*, Blackwell, 1990

Lee, V. and Das Gupta, P. (Eds), *Children's Cognitive and Language Development*, Open University, 1995

Meade, A. with Cubey, P., *Thinking Children*, New Zealand Council for Educational Research, 1996

Meadows, S., *The Child as Thinker*, Routledge, 1993

Mehler, J. and Dupoux, E., *What Infants Know*, Blackwell, 1994

Nutbrown, C., *Threads of Learning*, Paul Chapman, 1994

Smith, P. and Cowie, H., *Understanding Children's Development* (2nd edn), Blackwell, 1991

Thornton, S., *Children Solving Problems* (Developing Child series), Harvard UP, 1995

Tizard, B. and Hughes, M., *Young Children Learning*, Fontana, 1984

Wadsworth, B.J., *Piaget's Theory of Cognitive and Affective Development* (5th edn), Longman, 1996

Wood, D., *How Children Think and Learn*, Blackwell, 1988

Theorists

Jerome Bruner, Hans Eysenck, Ivan Pavlov, Jean Piaget, Burrhus Frederick Skinner, Lev Vygotsky, John Watson

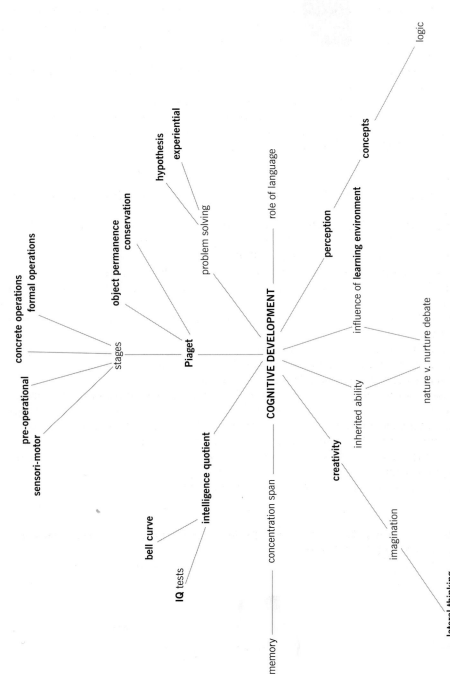

logic

hypothesis

experiential

object permanence
conservation

concrete operations
formal operations

role of language

problem solving

perception

influence of **learning environment**

concepts

stages

Piaget

pre-operational

sensori-motor

COGNITIVE DEVELOPMENT

nature v. nurture debate

inherited ability

intelligence quotient

bell curve

IQ tests

memory

concentration span

creativity

imagination

lateral thinking

8 Physical development and growth

Physical development describes the acquisition of skills, such as gross motor skills (e.g. running, sitting, and throwing) and fine motor skills (e.g. feeding, sewing and playing the piano). Growth is measurable: an increase in weight, height and head circumference. Potential growth is mainly genetically determined, although the environment will play its part. Better diet has resulted in taller and heavier people in most parts of the world. Babies are measured at birth, and this is used as a base line for subsequent monitoring. These measurements are recorded on percentile charts.

The acquisition of physical skills is dependent on the opportunity for practice and the encouragement of the carer. This acquisition is sequential and will not necessarily occur at the same time for all children. The development of gross motor skills starts with head control, and works down the body, the child learning to sit, crawl, pull up and walk. Fine motor skills are linked with vision and hand and eye co-ordination. These skills begin in the centre of the body, working outwards to the fingers, increasingly taking on more complex tasks.

All childcare practitioners need to be aware of the stages of development, regularly observing children in their care and implementing activities to encourage children to gain new skills. Evaluation of observations will allow children with developmental delay to be recognised and helped.

Resources
Barnes, P. (Ed), *Influencing Children's Development*, Blackwell and Open University, 1995
Bee, H., *Life Span Development*, Longman, 1998
Grossman, E., *Everyday Paediatrics*, Harcourt Brace, 1994
Hall, D., *Health for All Children*, Oxford Medical Publishers, 1989
Hall, J., *Gymnastic Activities for Infants*, A & E Black, 1996
Holt, K.S., *Child Development: Diagnosis and Assessment*, Butterworth Heinemann, 1994
Manchester City Council Education dept, *Education and Physical Education*, MCCE and JAS Publications, 1997
Mitchell, J., *Human Growth and Development: the childhood years*, Detselig Enterprises Ltd, 1990
Pearce, J., *Growth and Development*, Thorsons, 1994
Sherborne, V., *Developmental Movement for Children*, CUP, 1996
Sheridan, M., *From Birth to Five Years* (revised and updated by Frost, M. and Sharma, A.), Routledge, 1997

Addresses
The Child Growth Foundation, 2 Mayfield Road, London W4 1PW
Hyperactive Children's Support Group, 71 Whyke Lane, Chichester, West Sussex PO19 2LD

Theorist
Alfred Gesell

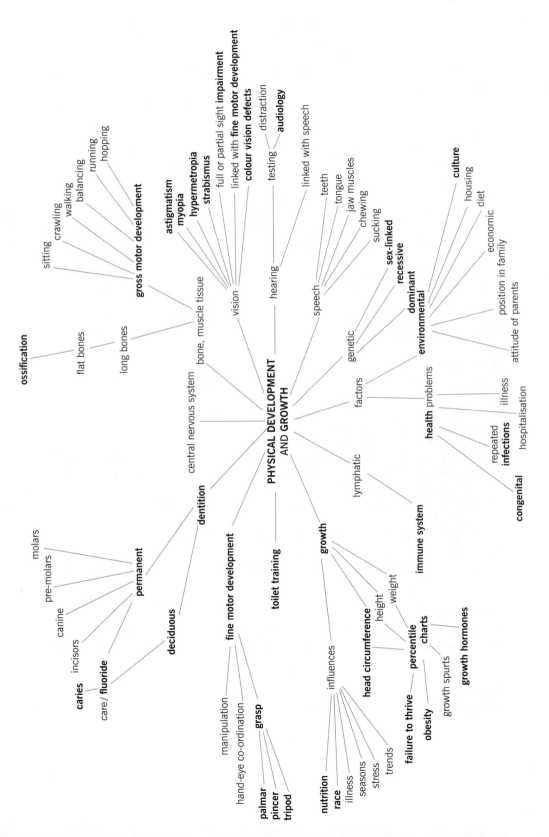

ossification

flat bones

long bones

sitting
crawling
walking
balancing
running
hopping

gross motor development

bone, muscle tissue

central nervous system

astigmatism
myopia
hypermetropia
strabismus
full or partial sight impairment
linked with **fine motor development**
colour vision defects
distraction
testing   **audiology**

vision

hearing

linked with speech

teeth
tongue
jaw muscles
chewing
sucking

speech

sex-linked
recessive
dominant

genetic

environmental

culture
housing
diet
economic
position in family
attitude of parents

factors

PHYSICAL DEVELOPMENT
AND GROWTH

health problems

illness
repeated
infections   hospitalisation

congenital

lymphatic

immune system

molars
pre-molars
canine
incisors
care / **fluoride**

caries

permanent

deciduous

dentition

fine motor development

manipulation
hand-eye co-ordination

palmar
pincer   **grasp**
tripod

toilet training

growth

height
weight

head circumference

percentile
charts

failure to thrive
obesity

growth hormones

growth spurts

influences

nutrition
race
illness
seasons
stress
trends

9 Challenging behaviour

You will meet many children in the course of your career who demonstrate behaviour which you will find challenging, covering a very wide spectrum. A child is neither 'naughty' nor 'good'. It is the behaviour that is unacceptable. As a professional worker, you will accept the behaviour and not take the aggression personally, never responding in kind, or saying that you do not like the child. This would make the child suffer low self-esteem. State calmly that you do not like the way he or she is behaving. For example, you might say that you do not like biting, or you do not think screaming is a good idea, and that maybe the child needs some time to think about the behaviour before he or she returns to their usual sunny self.

Your role is to discover the reason for the behaviour, and to do this you will find carrying out a series of observations, particularly time and event samples, invaluable. It is pointless to work out guidelines to help the child control his or her behaviour without the partnership of the parents. You will all need to communicate and work together with a consistent approach.

You will need a good understanding of age-appropriate behaviour. For example, a baby who cries for attention is behaving as a baby should, but the behaviour of a child of four who constantly screams for attention is not acceptable. Sometimes parents have unrealistic expectations of their children's behaviour, some being too strict and others over indulging. By working together, many difficulties can be sorted out.

Resources

Andreski, R. and Nicholls, S., *Managing Children's Behaviour*, Nursery World Publications, 1997

Bennathan, M. and Boxall, M., *Effective Intervention in Primary Schools*, David Fulton, 1996

Chazan, M. et al, *Helping Young Children with Behaviour Difficulties*, Croom Helm, 1983

Douglas, J., *Behaviour Problems in Young Children*, Routledge, 1989

Einon, D., *Child Behaviour*, Viking (Penguin), 1997

Laishley, J., *Working with Young Children*, Hodder & Stoughton, 1987

Leach, P., *No Smacking Guide to Good Behaviour*, Epoch, 1993

Richman, N. and Lansdown, R. (Eds), *Problems of Pre-school Children*, John Wiley and Sons, 1988

Roffey, S. and O'Rierdan, T., *Infant Class Behaviour Needs, Perspectives and Strategies*, David Fulton, 1996

Rutter, M., *Helping Troubled Children*, Penguin, 1975

Woolfson, R., *A–Z of Child Development*, Souvenir Press, 1993

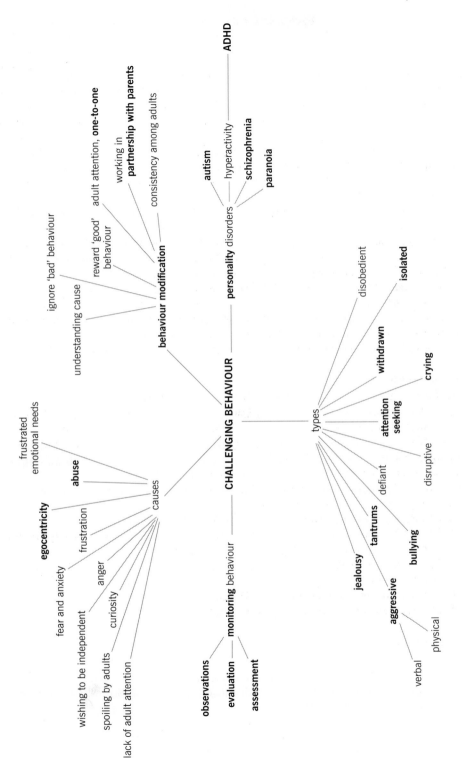

CHALLENGING BEHAVIOUR

causes
- **abuse**
- frustrated emotional needs
- **egocentricity**
- frustration
- fear and anxiety
- anger
- curiosity
- wishing to be independent
- spoiling by adults
- lack of adult attention

monitoring behaviour
- **observations**
- **evaluation**
- **assessment**

behaviour modification
- understanding cause
- ignore 'bad' behaviour
- reward 'good' behaviour
- adult attention, **one-to-one**
- working in **partnership with parents**
- consistency among adults

personality disorders
- **autism**
- hyperactivity — **ADHD**
- **schizophrenia**
- **paranoia**

types
- disobedient
- **isolated**
- **withdrawn**
- **crying**
- **attention seeking**
- disruptive
- defiant
- **bullying**
- **tantrums**
- **jealousy**
- **aggressive**
  - verbal
  - physical

10 Personal development

The personal development of a child is what makes him or her a unique human being. It relates to the spiritual, moral, aesthetic and creative development of the person. The capacity to develop creative skills, appreciate beauty, develop a conscience and to enjoy non-materialistic pursuits, if nurtured and encouraged, enables the child to grow into a holistic person, well rounded and caring for others.

With this in mind, the environment you create will be aesthetically pleasing, and the children's work will be valued and enhanced by being carefully mounted and displayed. The room will be clean and the home corner clothes and equipment spotless and well maintained. Where possible, natural materials will be chosen, rather than plastic resources. Books should be chosen for their illustrations as much as their anti-discriminatory text.

The place of religion in the curriculum is controversial. We live in a society that encompasses many faiths and it is important to find out as much as you can about the different religions, celebrating festivals, and respecting all beliefs.

It is thought that we are all born creative, and that this needs to be supported and encouraged from a young age, so as to foster a population that is creative in thought, imagination, the arts, and in the use of machinery. Children are born amoral, and learn from the family and from others a code of ethical behaviour that leads to the development of a conscience and the ability to know right from wrong.

Resources

Addis, I. and Spooner, S., *Assemblies*, Scholastic Publications, 1994
Barnes, P., (Ed.), *Personal, Social and Emotional Development of Children*, Blackwell and Open University, 1997
Breuillx, B. and Palmer, M., *Sainsbury's Religions of the World*, HarperCollins, 1993
Burgess, L. *Art Activities* (Bright Ideas for Early Years series), Scholastic Publications, 1994
Fountain, S., *Learning Together: Co-operative Games and Activities*, Centre for Global Education, 1990
Jenkins, J. *Contemporary Moral Issues* (3rd edn), Heinemann, 1997
Miller, J., *Never Too Young*, National Early Years Network/Save the Children, 1996
Makoff, J. and Duncan, L., *Display for all Seasons*, Belair Publications, 1996
Palmer, J., *Festivals*, Blueprint Series, Stanley Thornes, 1993
Perkiss, S., *Seeing, Making, Doing: creative development in the early years settings*, National Early Years Network, 1998
Rosen, M., *A World of Poetry*, Kingfisher, 1994

Addresses

Anti-Bullying Campaign, 101 Borough High Street, London SE1 9QQ. Telephone: 0171 378 1446. Website: http:www.com/homepages/anti-bullying
The National Society for Religious Education, 36 Causton Street, London SW1P 4AU. Telephone: 0171 932 1194

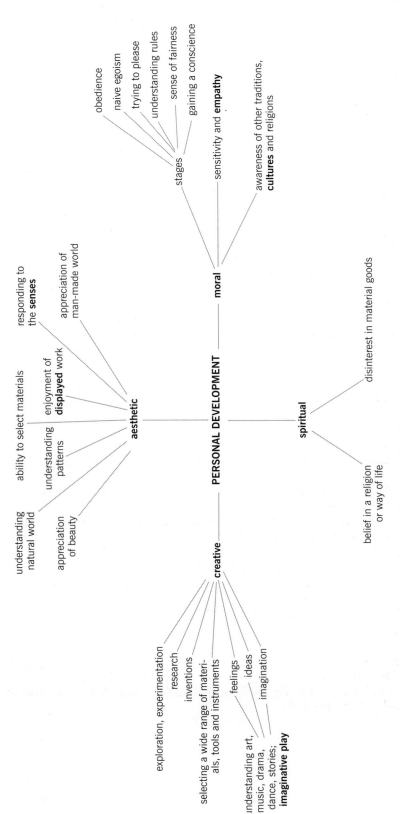

PERSONAL DEVELOPMENT

aesthetic
- understanding natural world
- ability to select materials
- responding to the **senses**
- appreciation of man-made world
- enjoyment of **displayed** work
- understanding patterns
- appreciation of beauty

moral
- stages
  - obedience
  - naive egoism
  - trying to please
  - understanding rules
  - sense of fairness
  - gaining a conscience
- sensitivity and **empathy**
- awareness of other traditions, **cultures** and religions

spiritual
- disinterest in material goods
- belief in a religion or way of life

creative
- exploration, experimentation
- research
- inventions
- selecting a wide range of materials, tools and instruments
- feelings
- ideas
- imagination
- understanding art, music, drama, dance, stories; **imaginative play**

11 Equal opportunities

It is essential that all childcare practitioners are totally committed to anti-discriminatory practices. No one should be discriminated against because of his or her race, gender, class, culture, age, religion, disability or sexual orientation. Children who are cared for without this commitment may develop negative feelings about themselves and their families, which would lead to a lack of self-esteem and inhibit their development.

All childcare settings should have policies making clear that these establishments are committed to equality of opportunity and you will need to familiarise yourself with these documents at the earliest opportunity. You must be ready to challenge prejudice and discriminatory practices.

Resources

Brown, B., *All Our Children*, BBC Books, 1993
Derman-Sparks, L., *Anti-bias Curriculum*, National Association for the Education of Young Children, Washington DC, 1989
Gajendra, K. et al, *Cultural Diversity and the Curriculum*, Vols. 1–4, Falmer Press
Hobart, C. and Frankel, J., *A Practical Guide to Working with Children* (2nd edn), Stanley Thornes, 1996
Malik, H., *A Practical Guide to Equal Opportunities*, Stanley Thornes, 1998
PLA, *Equal Chances* (2nd edn), 1996
Siraj-Blatchford, I., *The Early Years – Foundation for Racial Equality*, Trentham Books, 1994

Videos

Albany Video, *Being white and coffee coloured children*, Albany Video Distribution, Battersea Studios, Television Centre, Thackery Road, London SW8 3TW
Moonlight Films, *Marked for Life* (Mosaic series), BBC, 201 Wood Lane, London W12 7TS. Telephone 0181 752 5252
PLA, Wiltshire, *Building for the Future: equal opportunities for the under-fives through play in groups*. Telephone: 01380 726 440

Catalogues

Community Playthings, Robertsbridge, East Sussex, TN32 5DR. Freephone: 0800 387 457. Special furniture and equipment for children with disabilities.
Rompa, Goyt Side Road, Chesterfield, Derbyshire, S40 2PH. Telephone: 01645 211222. Products for children with hearing disabilities.

Leaflet

Peter White (UK version), *Playing fair – a parents guide to tackling discrimination*, The National Early Years Network and Save the Children, 1995

Addresses

Commission for Racial Equality, Elliott House, 10–12 Allington Street, London SE1 5EH. Telephone: 0171 828 7022
Early Years Trainers Anti-racist Network (EYTARN), PO Box 1870, London N12 8JQ. Telephone 0171 446 7056
Equal Opportunities Commission (EOC), Overseas House, Quay Street, Manchester M3 3HN. Telephone: 0161 833 9244
Save the Children Equality Learning Centre, The Resource Centre, 356 Holloway Road, London N7 6PA. Telephone: 0171 700 8127
Working Group Against Racism in Children's Resources, 460 Wandsworth Road, London SW8 3LX. Telephone: 0171 627 4594 (have a student information pack)

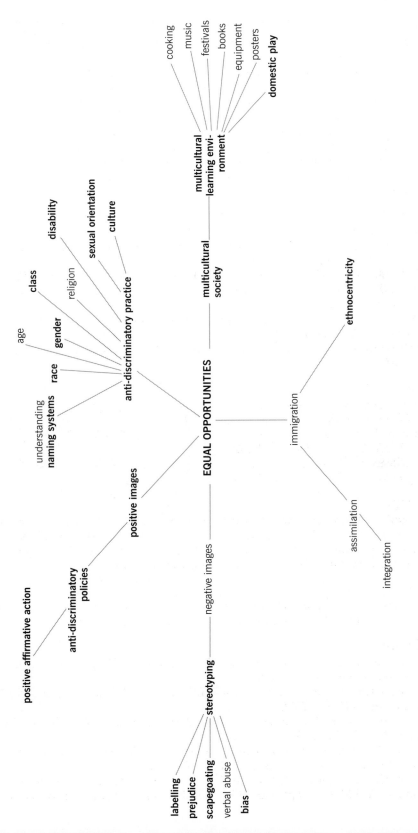

12 *Observations*

As a childcare practitioner, you will observe children in a knowledgeable and objective way on a regular basis, building up a record of observations and assessments which will lead to an understanding of the development and needs of children. These observations are focused and are carried out in order to plan for and assess children in a purposeful manner.

Developing these skills as a student will help you to understand your professional role and gain a valuable insight into what constitutes good practice.

Observations should be confidential, disclosure to anyone will depend on what is necessary to meet the needs of the child. It is important that you recognise the rights of parents, colleagues and children. Your observations should display empathy, respect and interest in all children and their families.

There is a variety of different ways of recording your observations, and you will become familiar with all the techniques in many different situations. Whatever employment you finally choose, observations are integral to your work and will enrich your practice.

Resources

Beaty, J., *Observing the Development of Young Children* (4th edn), Prentice Hall, 1998

Blenkin, G. and Kelly, A. (Eds), *Assessment in Early Childhood Education*, Paul Chapman, 1992

Clemson, D. and Clemson, W., *The Really Practical Guide to Primary Assessment* (2nd edn), Stanley Thornes, 1996

Drummond, M., *Assessing Children's Learning*, David Fulton Press, 1993

Drummond, M. and Nutbrown, C., 'Observing and assessing young children' in Pugh, G. (Ed.), *Contemporary Issues in the Early Years*, NCB/ Paul Chapman, 1992

Drummond, M., Rouse, D. and Pugh, G., *Making Assessment Work*, NES Arnold/NCB, 1992

Fawcett, M., *Learning Through Child Observation*, Jessica Kingsley, 1996

Hobart, C. and Frankel, J., *A Practical Guide to Child Observation*, Stanley Thornes, 1994

Hutchins, V., *Tracking Significant Achievement in the Early Years*, Hodder & Stoughton, 1996

Miller, L. et al, *Closely Observed Infants*, G. Duckworth and Co Ltd, 1989

Quilham, S., *Child Watching; a parents guide to body language*, Ward Lock, 1994

Sylva, K. et al, *Childwatching at Playgroup and Nursery School*, Grant McIntyre, 1980

Wolfendale, S., *Baseline Assessment*, Trentham Books, 1993

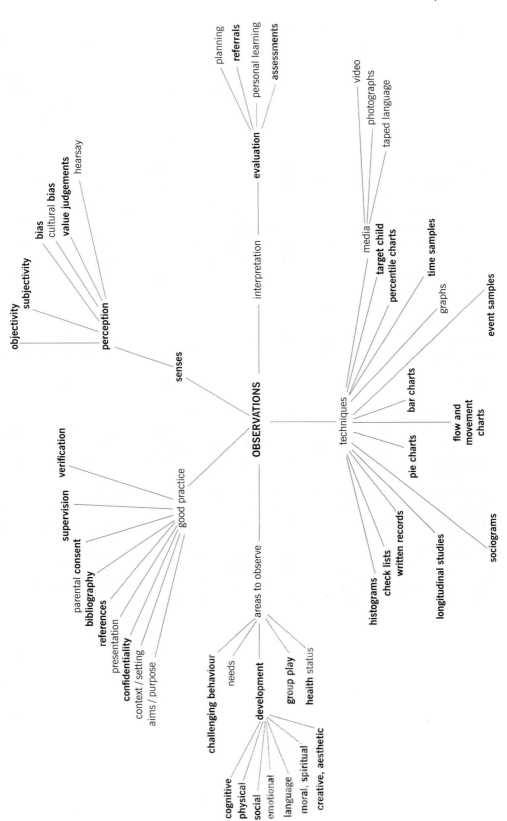

planning
referrals
personal learning
assessments
evaluation

bias
cultural bias
value judgements
hearsay

video
photographs
taped language

objectivity
subjectivity

interpretation

perception

media
target child
percentile charts
time samples

senses

graphs

OBSERVATIONS

event samples

techniques

verification

bar charts

supervision

good practice

**flow and
movement
charts**

parental **consent**
bibliography
references
presentation
confidentiality
context / setting
aims / purpose

pie charts

areas to observe

histograms
check lists
written records

challenging behaviour
needs

sociograms

group play
health status

longitudinal studies

development

cognitive
physical
social
emotional
language
moral, spiritual
creative, aesthetic

13 Pre-school provision

Before children attend school, they may be cared for in many diverse settings. Up to the age of two most children are cared for in the home. Even so, there are many specialist classes provided for them, where they can extend their skills in art, music, swimming and gymnastics. For this young age group there are also parent and toddler groups and drop in centres. In all these places the child must be accompanied by an adult.

Children may be looked after in the home by their parents, a nanny, another member of the extended family, an au pair or a mother's help. They may go to another home and be looked after by a registered child-minder.

For some children, daycare may be provided, either by the local authority, a voluntary group or within the private sector. Most children will be two years of age or older, but there is provision for a small number of babies.

From two and a half to three years, the choice widens. The educational establishments provide nursery classes and nursery schools, and the Pre-school Learning Alliance sponsor many pre-schools throughout the country. Many children continue to attend private groups, partly because there is not enough provision for all the children under the state system. Some places are part-time, and some are sessional. Even if the provision is full-time, it often fails to meet the need of working parents. In some parts of the country, there is very little provision for three year olds and many four year olds attend the infant school early, which is not always appropriate. The ratio of adult to children is much larger, and the freedom to work on one's own is often curtailed.

Resources

Andreski, R. and Nicholls, S., *Setting Standards*, Nursery World Publications, 1995
Curtis, A., *Early Childhood Education Explained*, OMEP, 1994
Hennessy, et al., *Children and Daycare*, Paul Chapman, 1992
Kozak, M., *Daycare for Kids*, Daycare Trust, 1989
McQuail, S. and Pugh, G., *Effective Organisation of Early Childhood Services*, NCB, 1995
Moss, P. and Penn, H., *Transforming Nursery Education*, Paul Chapman, 1996
Petrie, P., *Play and Care*, HMSO, 1994
Robson, B., *Pre-school Provision for Children with Special Needs*, Cassell, 1989
Smith, C., *A Guide to Daycare Services and Standards under the Children Act, 1989*, Early Years Network/VOLCUF, 1991
Working for Child Care: a practical guide to workplace nurseries, Working for Child Care, 1993

Addresses

Black Child Care Network, 17 Brownhill Road, Catford, London SE6
Daycare Trust, 4 Wild Court, London WC2B 4AU. Telephone: 0171 405 5617
National Childminding Association, 8 Masons Hill, Bromley, Kent BR2 9EY. Telephone: 0181 464 6164
National Children's Bureau, 8 Wakely Street, London EC1V 7QE. Telephone: 0171 843 6000. Website: www.ncb.org.UK
National Early Years Network, 77 Holloway Road, Islington, London N7 8J2. Telephone: 0171 607 9573. Website: www.ncb.org.UK
Pre-school Learning Alliance, 69 King's Cross Road, London WC1X 9LL. Telephone: 0171 833 0991

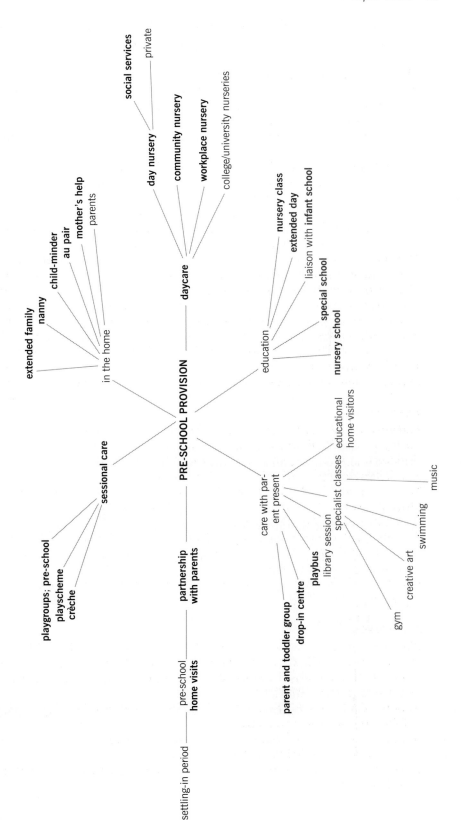

PRE-SCHOOL PROVISION

in the home
- extended family
- nanny
- child-minder
- au pair
- mother's help
- parents

daycare
- day nursery
- community nursery
- workplace nursery
- college/university nurseries
- social services
- private

education
- nursery class
- extended day
- liaison with infant school
- special school
- nursery school

sessional care
- playgroups; pre-school
- playscheme
- crèche

partnership with parents
- pre-school home visits
- settling-in period

care with parent present
- parent and toddler group
- drop-in centre
- playbus
- library session
- specialist classes
- educational home visitors
- gym
- creative art
- swimming
- music

14 Play

Play has been called 'children's work', and is an integral part of the daily life and the promotion of all-round development. Through play, the child experiences life and learns to understand the world and his or her place in it.

The baby plays from birth, the first 'toy' being the mother's breast. From this first stage, play develops through several stages to co-operative games with complicated rules.

There are many different types of play, indoor and out, structured and spontaneous. Adults should avoid intervening too frequently and attempting to impose too rigid a structure on children's imaginative play. By interaction with the children, the adult can enrich the play, as long as this is done sensitively, based on observation and assessment of the child's need.

Resources

Bruce, T., *Helping Young Children to Play*, Hodder & Stoughton , 1996
    Time to Play in Early Childhood Education, Hodder & Stoughton, 1991
Cohen, D., *The Development of Play* (2nd edn), Routledge, 1993
Garvey, C., *Play* (2nd edn) (Developing Child series), Fontana Press, 1991
Matterson, E., *Play with a Purpose for the Under Sevens* (3rd edn), Penguin, 1989
Melville, S., *Gender Matters*, Playboard, 1994
Moyles, J., *Just Playing*, OUP, 1989
    (Ed.), *The Excellence of Play*, OUP, 1994
Sheridan, M., *Spontaneous Play in Early Childhood*, Routledge, 1977

Catalogues

Galt Toys, Brookfield Road, Cheadle, Cheshire SK8 2PN. Telephone: 0161 428 9111
NES Arnold, Ludlow Hill Road, West Bridgeford, Nottingham NG 6HD. Telephone:
    01602 452 201

Addresses

Childsplay (multicultural toy shop), 112 Tooting High Street, London SW17 0RR.
    Telephone: 0171 828 7088. Dr Toy Website: http://www.drtoy.com/
National Association of Toy and Leisure Libraries, 68 Churchway, London NW1 1LT.
    Telephone: 0171 387 4592

Theorist
Frederick Froebel

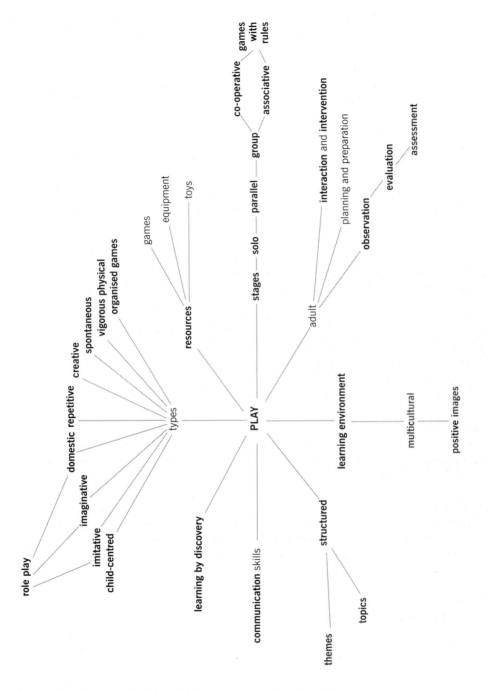

15 *Early years education*

Early years refers to the education of children from birth to eight years old. The implementation of the National Curriculum has made specific demands on the education of young children, and this has influenced the curriculum of the children in the pre-school and in the infant school, so that the 'desirable outcomes' are achieved.

There has been a shift from the emphasis on caring for children's physical, social and emotional needs to a more cognitive approach. Children are assessed at five and again at seven. The day is more structured to ensure ample time for the children to learn basic skills.

Resources

Abbott, L. and Rodger, R., *Quality Education in the Early Years*, Open University, 1994
Allebone, B., *Number Time*, BBC Education, 1997
Anning, A. (Ed.), *A National Curriculum for the Early Years*, OUP, 1995
Bruce, T., *Early Childhood Education*, Hodder & Stoughton, 1997
Cockburn, Anne D., *Beginning Teaching*, Paul Chapman, 1992
Curtis, A., *A Curriculum for the Pre-school Child*, NFER/Nelson, 1986
David, T. (Ed.), *Working Together for Young Children*, Routledge, 1994
Dowling, M., *Education 3–5* (2nd edn), Paul Chapman, 1992
Drummond, M.J., *Assessing Children's Learning*, David Fulton, 1994
Edgington, M., *The Nursery Teacher in Action* (2nd edn), Paul Chapman, 1998
Finch, S., *Computers in Early Years Settings*, National Early Years Network, 1997
Gura, P., *Resources for Early Learning: Children, Adults and Stuff*, Hodder & Stoughton, 1996
Hughes, M., *Children and Number*, Blackwell, 1986
Kennedy, J. (Ed.), *Primary Science*, Routledge, 1997
Kerry, T. and Tollitt, J., *Teaching Infants*, Stanley Thornes, 1992
Neaum, S. and Tallack, J., *Good Practice in Implementing the Pre-school Curriculum*, Stanley Thornes, 1997
Pluckrose, H., *Starting School: the vital years*, Simon & Schuster, 1993
Nutbrown, C., *Threads of Thinking*, Paul Chapman, 1994
Pascal, C. and Bertram, T., *Effective Early Learning*, Hodder & Stoughton, 1997
Richards, R., Collis, M. and Kincaid, D., *An Early Start to Science*, Simon & Schuster, 1987
Whitebread, D., *Teaching and Learning*, Routledge, 1996

Videos

OFSTED, *Literacy Matters* and *Teachers Count*, £11.75 each. Telephone: 01937 5411010

Addresses

Advisory Centre for Education (ACE), 18 Aberdeen Studios, 22 Highbury Grove, London N5 2DQ. Telephone: 0171 354 8318. Website: www/ace/ed.org.UK
British Association for Early Childhood Education (BAECE), 111 City View House, 463 Bethnal Green Road, London E2 9QY. Telephone: 0171 739 7594
Department for Education and Employment, Sanctuary Buildings, Great Smith Street, London SW1P 3BT. Telephone: 0171 925 5000
High Scope, Copperfield House, 190–192 Maple Road, London SE20 8HT. Telephone: 0181 676 0220
National Campaign for Nursery Education (NCNE), BCM Box 6216, London WC1N 3XX

Educationalists

Frederick Froebel, Susan Isaacs, Maria Montessori, Margaret and Rachel Macmillan, Rudolph Steiner

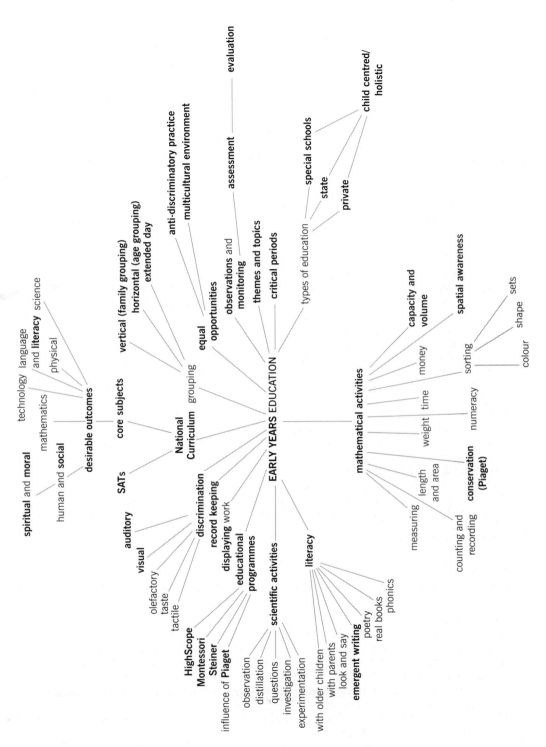

EARLY YEARS EDUCATION

desirable outcomes
- spiritual and moral
- human and social
- technology
- language and literacy
- science
- mathematics
- physical

core subjects

National Curriculum

grouping
- vertical (family grouping)
- horizontal (age grouping)
- extended day

equal opportunities
- anti-discriminatory practice
- multicultural environment

observations and monitoring
- themes and topics
- critical periods

assessment — evaluation

types of education
- special schools
- state
- private
- child centred/ holistic

SATs

discrimination
- auditory
- visual
- olefactory
- taste
- tactile

record keeping
displaying work

educational programmes
- influence of Piaget
- HighScope
- Montessori
- Steiner

scientific activities
- observation
- distillation
- questions
- investigation
- experimentation
- with older children
- with parents
- look and say

literacy
- emergent writing
- poetry
- real books
- phonics

mathematical activities
- capacity and volume
- spatial awareness
- money
- time
- weight
- length and area
- numeracy
- conservation (Piaget)
- counting and recording
- measuring
- sorting
- sets
- shape
- colour

16 Activities with children

When working with young children, you need to remember that all activities should promote the children's all-round development. You should provide a range of activities that are both well planned and well prepared. You must check that all the material you may need is in stock, and that you have sufficient time and space to carry out the activity satisfactorily.

Consultation is necessary with other members of the team, so that the requirements of the National Curriculum are fulfilled and desirable learning outcomes are achieved.

Through your observations, you will be able to plan your activities with the children's developmental needs in mind. There may be occasions when you feel that unstructured and spontaneous activities will be fun for all concerned, and allow children to use their imagination and develop close peer relationships. There are very few activities in the pre-school years that do not have some value. The important point is that you are aware of the value of the work you are planning and preparing, and that you take time to evaluate the outcomes of the activities.

All activities should be age appropriate and reflect our diverse multicultural society. All the children should have equal access to all the activities.

Resources

Bright Ideas for Early Years Series and Bright Ideas Series, Scholastic Publications Ltd

Brown, B., *All Our Children*, BBC Educational Publishing, 1993

Fountain, S., *Learning Together: Co-operative Games and Activities*, Centre for Global Education, 1990

Goldschmied, E. and Jackson, S., *People Under Three*, Routledge, 1994

Hall, N. and Abbot, L. (Eds), *Play in the Primary Curriculum*, Hodder & Stoughton, 1994

Hobart, C. and Frankel, J., *A Practical Guide to Activities for Young Children*, Stanley Thornes, 1995

Holtzman, M., *The Language of Children*, Blackwell, 1997

Terzian, A., *The Kids Multicultural Artbook*, Williams, 1993

The Best Guide to Days Out Ever, Best Guides Ltd, 1997

Tizzard, B. and Hughes, M., *Young Children Learning*, Fontana, 1984

Catalogue

Criteria for Play Equipment, Community Playthings, Robertsbridge, East Sussex TN32 5DR. Telephone: 0800 387 457

Addresses

Best Guides Ltd, PO Box 427, Northampton NN2 7YJ. Telephone: 01604 711 994

The Letterbox Library, Unit 2D Leroy House, 436 Essex Road, London N1 3QP. Telephone: 0171 226 1633

National Association of Toy and Leisure Libraries, 68 Churchway, London NW1 1LT. Telephone: 0171 387 4592

Save the Children Equality Learning Centre, 356 Holloway Road, London N7 6PA. Telephone: 0171 700 8127

Scholastic Publications Ltd, Freepost CV1034, Westfield Road, Southern Leamington Spa, Warwickshire CV33 0BR

The Working Group Against Racism in Children's Resources, 460 Wandsworth Road, London SW8 3LX. Telephone: 0171 627 4594

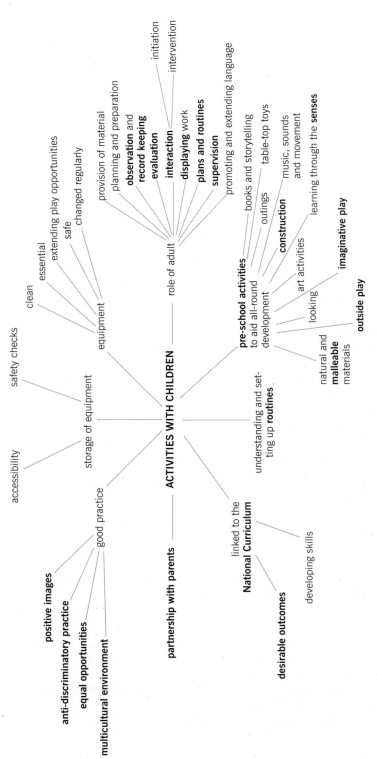

17 Partnership with parents

The Children Act, 1989, has reinforced the importance of childcare practitioners working in partnership with parents of young children. You will find yourself involved with parents at several levels: on a day-to-day basis in your establishment, when parents deliver and collect children and perhaps stay to help from time to time; parent teacher associations, governing bodies and management committees, perhaps linked to fund-raising; involving parents on outings and contributing their special skills to the group; and encouraging parents to help their children develop new skills, such as reading with them at home. If you are working as a nanny, you will be caring for the children in partnership with your employer. If you are employed in a private establishment, there is increasing emphasis on the parent as a customer and purchaser of care for their child.

You may find yourself working with parents who have neglected or abused their children. In this difficult situation, you will need to draw on your knowledge of child protection issues, your professionalism and the support of your colleagues.

Resources

Ball, M., *Consulting with Parents*, National Early Years Network, 1997
Bastiani, J., *Working with Parents* (A Whole School Approach), Windsor/NFER/Nelson, 1989
EYTARN, Partnership with Parents: an Anti-discriminatory Approach, EYTARN, 1997
Hobart, C. and Frankel, J., *A Practical Guide to Working with Parents*, Stanley Thornes, 1999
  Good Practice in Child Protection, Stanley Thornes, 1998
Hyder, T. et al, *On Equal Terms*, National Early Years Network/Save the Children, 1997
Kenway, P., *Working with Parents*, Save the Children/Reading and Language Information Unit, University of Reading, 1994
Pugh, G. et al., *Confident Parents, Confident Children*, NCB, 1994
Pugh, G. and De'Ath, E., *Working Towards Partnership in the Early Years*, NCB, 1989

Addresses

Effective Parenting, 117 Corringham Road, London NW11 7DL. Telephone: 0181 458 8404
Exploring Parenthood, 4 Ivory Parade, Treadgold Street, London W11 4BP. Telephone: 0171 221 4471
Home Start, UK, 2 Salisbury Road, Leicester LE1 7QR. Telephone: 0116 233 9955
National Confederation of Parent/Teacher Associations, 2 Ebbsfleet Industrial Estate, Stonebridge Road, Gravesend, Kent DA11 9DT
Parent Line, Endway House, The Endway, Hadleigh, Benfleet, Essex SS7 2AN. Telephone: 01702 554782
Parent Network/Parent Infant Project, 44–46 Caversham Road, London NW5. Telephone: 0171 485 8535
Parenting, Education and Support Forum, 8 Wakely Street, London EC1V 7QE. Telephone: 0171 843 6099

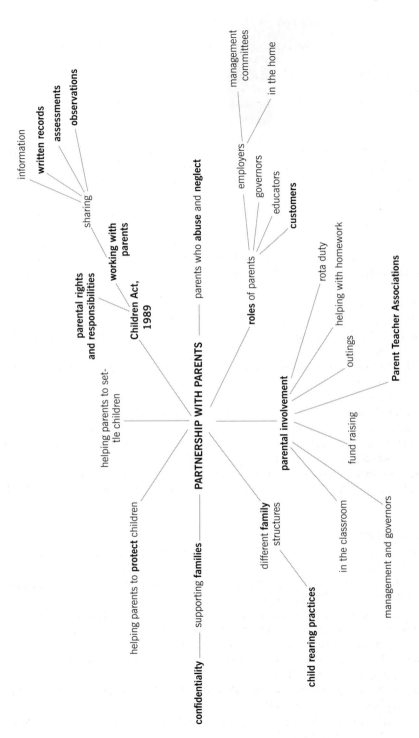

information
written records
assessments
observations

sharing

management
committees

in the home

employers

governors

educators

customers

**parental rights
and responsibilities**

**working with
parents**

**Children Act,
1989**

roles of parents

rota duty

helping parents to set-
tle children

helping with homework

PARTNERSHIP WITH PARENTS ———— parents who **abuse** and **neglect**

outings

parental involvement

helping parents to **protect** children

fund raising

Parent Teacher Associations

confidentiality ———— supporting families

different **family**
structures

in the classroom

child rearing practices

management and governors

18 Safety

In order to discover and learn about the world, children need to be able to explore their environment. They must be protected and live and work in an environment that has been made safe. Knowledge of the stages of development will ensure that you are aware of hazards that may present a risk to children at certain ages and stages. For example, a bottle of bleach on the floor will not present a risk to a baby of two months, but could spell death to an inquisitive child of nine months. Anyone working with children should undertake a recognised first aid course, and ensure that they constantly update this qualification.

Danger is all around us. If you are working in the family setting, one of the first things you will do is to check the house and garden for possible hazards and make sure that the family car is well maintained and has the necessary restraints and seat belts. Personal hygiene, and cleanliness in the kitchen is essential, so as to guard against the dangers of food poisoning. Working in an establishment, you will be aware of health and safety procedures and carrying out regular checks of all equipment both inside and out of doors. You will know the location of the first aid box and what to do in any emergency.

You will present yourself as a good role model to children and ensure that you help them develop an awareness of possible hazards, and how to protect themselves. For example, when going on an outing, you will point out to the children the best and safest place to cross a busy street.

Resources

Child Accident Prevention Trust, *Accident Prevention in Daycare and Play Settings*, CAPT, 1994

First Aid for Children – Fast, Dorling Kindersley in association with British Red Cross, 1994

Levene, S., *Play it Safe: the complete guide to child accident prevention*, BBC Books, 1992

Wolfe, L., *Safe and Sound*, Hodder & Stoughton, 1993

Addresses

Child Accident Prevention Trust (CAPT), Clerks Court, 18/20 Farringdon Lane, London EC1R 3AU. Telephone 0171 608 3828. Website: www.qub.ac.uk/cm/eph/capt/index.htm

Health and Safety Executive, Information Service, Broad Lane, Sheffield S3 7HQ and PO Box 1999, Sudbury, Suffolk CO10 6FS. Telephone 0114 289 2345

Royal Society for the Prevention of Accidents (RoSPA), Cannon House, The Priory, Queensway, Birmingham B4 6BS. Telephone: 0121 248 2000

St John Ambulance National Headquarters, 1 Grosvenor Crescent, London SW1X 7EF. Telephone 0171 235 5231

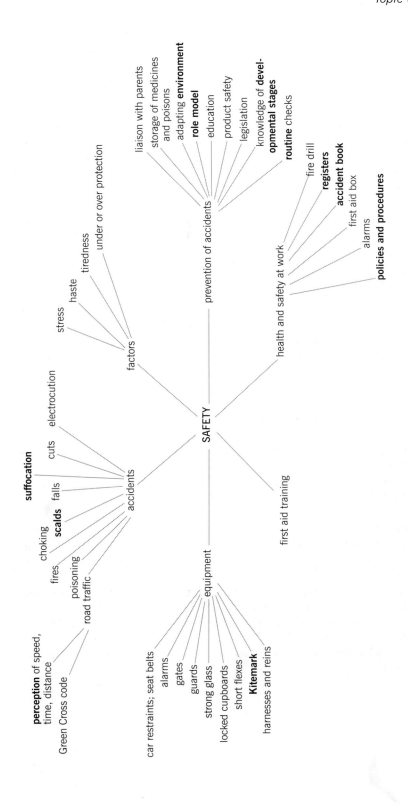

SAFETY

factors
- stress
  - haste
  - tiredness
- under or over protection

accidents
- electrocution
- cuts
- falls
- **scalds**
- **suffocation**
- choking
- fires
- poisoning
- road traffic
  - **perception** of speed, time, distance
  - Green Cross code

equipment
- car restraints; seat belts
- alarms
- gates
- guards
- strong glass
- locked cupboards
- short flexes
- **Kitemark**
- harnesses and reins

first aid training

prevention of accidents
- liaison with parents
- storage of medicines and poisons
- adapting **environment**
- **role model**
- education
- product safety
- legislation
- knowledge of **developmental stages**
- **routine** checks

health and safety at work
- fire drill
- **registers**
- **accident book**
- first aid box
- alarms
- **policies and procedures**

19 Child protection

Children have a right to be protected against abuse, both inside and outside the home, and you, as a childcare practitioner will need to be clear about your role in this stressful area. You will learn how to identify children who may be at risk, to recognise the signs and symptoms of abuse and to understand the procedures and policies that are in place to protect children. Your role is not to investigate abuse and neglect.

You may have to work with children who have suffered abuse or neglect, and have to communicate with their families. You will attempt to instil in all children skills that will help them protect themselves. You will need a thorough knowledge of all the agencies who work together to ensure our children are safe.

You may find yourself having to attend child protection conferences where your recorded observations will be invaluable, and your contribution to the child protection plan will be appreciated.

Resources

Alsop, P. and McCaffrey, T., *How to Cope with Childhood Stress*, NSPCC, 1996
Axline, V., *Play Therapy* (2nd edn), Churchill Livingstone, 1989
Cattanach, A., *Play Therapy with Abused Children*, Jessica Kingsley, 1993
Department of Health, *Messages From Research*, HMSO, 1995
Elliot, M., *Keeping Safe: a Practical Guide to Talking to Children*, Coronet Books, 1994
Hobart, C. and Frankel, J., *Good Practice in Child Protection*, Stanley Thornes, 1998
Lyon, C., and de Cruz, P., *Child Abuse*, Jordan, 1993
Pugh, G. and Hallaves, A., *Child Protection in Early Childhood Services*, National Children's Bureau, 1994
Walker, A., *Possessing the Secret of Joy*, Jonathan Cape, 1992
Whitney, B., *Child Protection for Teachers in Schools*, Kogan Page, 1996

Addresses

British Association for the Study and Prevention of Child Abuse and Neglect, 10 Priory Street, York YO1 1E2. Telephone: 01904 613605
ChildLine, 2nd Floor Royal Mail Buildings, Studd Street, London N1 0QW. Telephone: 0171 239 1000 (for children 0800 1111)
End Physical Punishment of Children (EPOCH), 77 Holloway Road, London N7 8JZ. Telephone: 0171 750 0627
Kidscape, 152 Buckingham Palace Road, London SW1W 9TR. Telephone: 0171 730 3300. Website: www.solnet.co.UK/kidscape/
NSPCC, 42 Curtain Road, London EC2A 3NH. Telephone: 0171 825 2500 (helpline 0800 800 500). Website: www.nspcc.org.UK
Save the Children Fund, 17 Grove Lane, London SE5 8RD. Telephone: 0171 703 5400

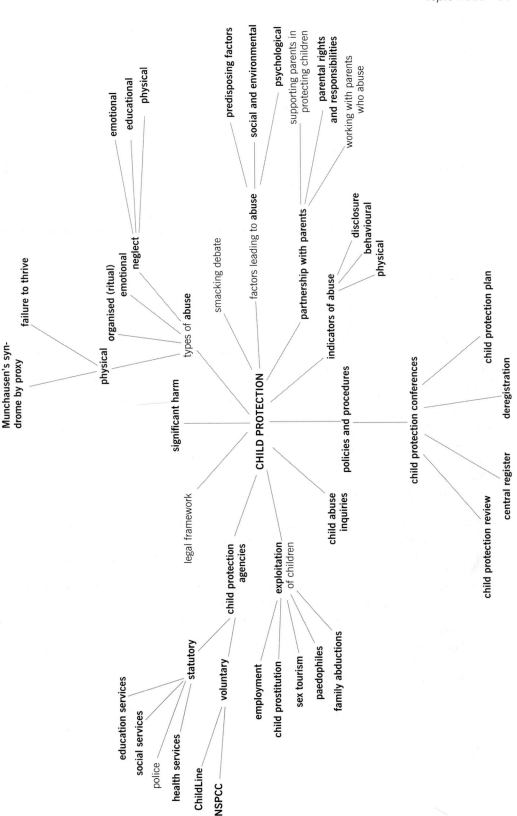

CHILD PROTECTION

Munchausen's syn-
drome by proxy

failure to thrive

physical

types of **abuse**

emotional
educational
physical

neglect

organised (ritual)
emotional
physical

smacking debate

predisposing factors

social and environmental

psychological

factors leading to abuse

supporting parents in
protecting children

**parental rights
and responsibilities**

working with parents
who abuse

partnership with parents

disclosure
behavioural
physical

indicators of abuse

significant harm

legal framework

**child protection
agencies**

education services
social services
police
health services
ChildLine
NSPCC

statutory

voluntary

employment
child prostitution
sex tourism
paedophiles
family abductions

exploitation
of children

child abuse
inquiries

policies and procedures

child protection conferences

child protection review

central register

deregistration

child protection plan

20 Food and nutrition

It is important for the childcare practitioner to have a good understanding of nutrition and how to provide a well-balanced diet for the children in his or her care. A healthy nutritious diet plays a large part in promoting health, and in ensuring optimum development. The childcare practitioner acts as a role model in developing healthy eating patterns and will encourage children to try many different types of food from around the world.

Cooking with children is not only an emotional and intellectual activity, but establishes good habits and understanding of nutrition. Children are able to see for themselves that fresh food can be cooked in the home, and does not have to be packaged or tinned. Parents are often pleased to be involved in organising cooking sessions and in being consulted in the cooking of various ethnic dishes.

During the process of home visiting and settling a child into a nursery setting, the parents will inform you of any special dietary requirements. You will need to have a good knowledge of special diets and understand why these are necessary.

Resources

Dare, A. and O'Donovan, M., *A Practical Guide to Child Nutrition*, Stanley Thornes, 1996

Duft, Elizabeth, 'On the sugar trail' in *Nursery World*, 29.9.94; 'Vitamins' in *Nursery World*, 6.10.94; 'Fat in children's diets' in *Nursery World*, 13.10.94

Edwards, N., *Food*, Messages Series, A & C Black (Publishers Ltd), 1995

Hill, S.E., *More than Rice and Peas*, Food Commission, 1990

HMSO, *The Manual of Nutrition* (10th edn), HMSO, 1995

Jones, A., *Nutrition and Cookery for Nursery Nurses*, Longman, 1988

Sandy, D., *Food in Care*, Macmillan Caring Series, 1996

Steward Treswell, A., *ABC of Nutrition* (2nd edn), BMJ, 1992

Thompson, J. (Ed.), *Nutritional Requirements of Infants and Young Children*, Blackwell Scientific, 1998

Tull, A., *Food and Nutrition* (3rd edn), OUP, 1996

Whiting, M. and Lobstein, T., *The Nursery Food Book*, Edward Arnold, 1992

Wilkins, V. *Cookery Cards for Children*, Tamarind Books, 1995

Addresses

The British Diabetic Association, 10 Queen Anne Street, London W1M 0BD. Website: www.diabetic.org.UK

Child Growth Foundation, 2 Mayfield Avenue, Chiswick, London W4 1PW

The Coeliac Society, PO Box 220, High Wycombe, Bucks HP11 2HY

Food Commission, 102 Gloucester Place, London W1H 3DA

School Meals Campaign, PO Box 402, London WC1H 9TZ

The Vegetarian Society, Parkdale, Dunham Road, Altrincham, Cheshire WA14 4QG

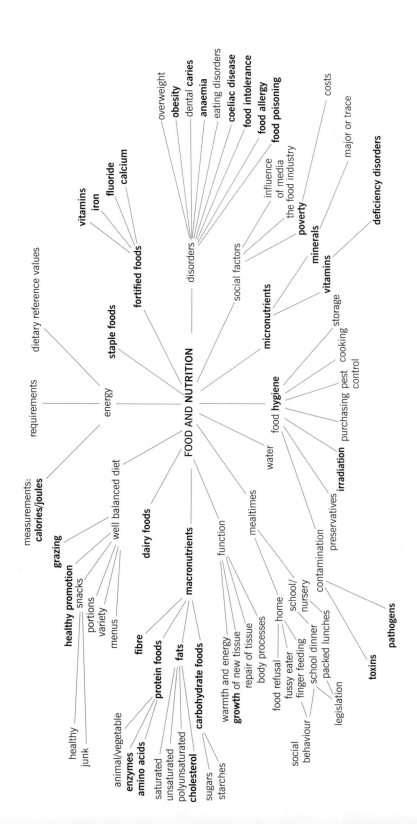

FOOD AND NUTRITION

energy
 requirements
 dietary reference values
 measurements:
 calories/joules

healthy promotion
 grazing
 snacks
 portions
 variety
 menus
 well balanced diet
 healthy
 junk

staple foods

fortified foods
 vitamins
 iron
 fluoride
 calcium

disorders
 overweight
 obesity
 dental **caries**
 anaemia
 eating disorders
 coeliac disease
 food intolerance
 food allergy
 food poisoning

social factors
 influence
 of media
 the food industry
 poverty
 costs

micronutrients
 minerals
 vitamins
 major or trace
 deficiency disorders

dairy foods

macronutrients
 fibre
 protein foods
 enzymes
 amino acids
 animal/vegetable
 fats
 saturated
 unsaturated
 polyunsaturated
 cholesterol
 carbohydrate foods
 sugars
 starches

function
 warmth and energy
 growth of new tissue
 repair of tissue
 body processes

mealtimes
 home
 school/
 nursery
 food refusal
 fussy eater
 finger feeding
 school dinner
 packed lunches
 social
 behaviour
 legislation

water

food **hygiene**
 storage
 cooking
 pest
 control
 purchasing
 irradiation
 preservatives
 contamination
 toxins
 pathogens

21 Prevention of infection

Infection is the most common cause of illness in young children and, if frequent, can cause developmental delay and impede growth. As a childcare practitioner it is important that you know the different types of infection, how they are communicated to others, and how to prevent the spread of infection.

Infection can range from the common cold to meningitis and as you gain experience you will find it easier to diagnose the symptoms of the illness. If you are in charge of a child who suddenly becomes ill you must contact the parents and if you have any concerns you must seek medical advice. You should encourage parents to participate in immunisation programmes so as to reduce incidence of childhood diseases, which can be very dangerous.

Resources

Department of Health, *Immunisation Against Infectious Diseases*, HMSO (updated every year)
    Infectious Diseases in Schools: prevention and control, HMSO, 1991
Health Education Authority, *Childhood Diseases Haven't Died: Children Have*, HMSO
Immunisation Fact Sheets, HMSO, 1997
Hogg, C., *Living Positively*, NCB, 1996
Nicoll, A. (Ed.), *Manual of Infections and Immunisations in Children*, Oxford Medical Publications, 1989
Noel, G., et al, *Paediatric Infectious Diseases*, Johns Hopkins University Press, 1997

Video

You Could Make the Difference (encouraging parents to immunise their children) produced by the Health Education Authority.

Addresses

Children with AIDS Charity (CWAC), 2nd Floor, 111 High Holborn, London WC1V 6JS. Telephone: 0171 242 3883. Website: www.cwac.demon.co.UK
Health Education Authority, Hamilton House, Mabledon Place, London WC1 9TX
HMSO, Publication Centre, 51 Nine Elms Lane, London SW8 5DR. Telephone: 0171 873 0011
Terence Higgins Trust, 52–54 Gray's Inn Road, London WC1X 8JU. Telephone: 0171 831 0330. Website: www.tht.org.UK

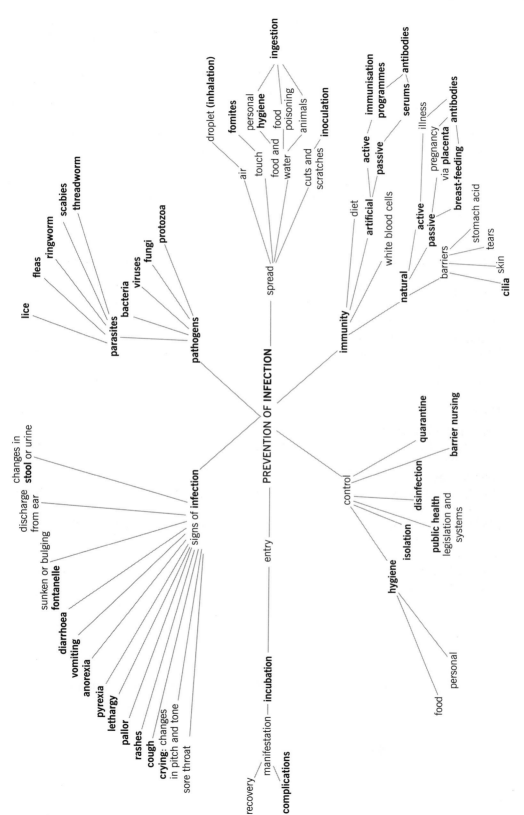

PREVENTION OF INFECTION

pathogens
- parasites
  - lice
  - fleas
  - ringworm
  - scabies
  - threadworm
- bacteria
- viruses
- fungi
- protozoa

spread
- air
  - droplet (inhalation)
- touch
  - fomites
  - personal hygiene
- food and water
  - ingestion
    - food poisoning
    - animals
  - inoculation
  - cuts and scratches
  - inoculation

immunity
- diet
- white blood cells
- artificial
  - active
  - passive
  - immunisation programmes
  - serums
  - antibodies
- natural
  - active
    - illness
  - passive
    - pregnancy
    - via placenta
    - breast-feeding
    - antibodies
  - barriers
    - stomach acid
    - tears
    - skin
    - cilia

control
- quarantine
- barrier nursing
- disinfection
- isolation
- public health legislation and systems
- hygiene
  - food
  - personal

entry
- manifestation
- incubation
- recovery
- complications

signs of infection
- changes in **stool** or urine
- discharge from ear
- sunken or bulging **fontanelle**
- **diarrhoea**
- **vomiting**
- anorexia
- **pyrexia**
- **lethargy**
- **pallor**
- **rashes**
- **cough**
- **crying**: changes in pitch and tone
- sore throat

22 *The sick child*

You have a key role in working with sick children, in observing, recording and reporting symptoms to parents and medical staff. You may have to provide basic nursing care in the home setting being responsible for medication, physical care, emotional support, and appropriate play activities during convalescence.

You will appreciate that the child may regress, both in behaviour and in cognitive skills during periods of illness.

In any area of employment, you may find yourself preparing a child for a planned hospital admission, in partnership with the parents. As some children in your care may be admitted to hospital in an emergency, it is important that an area of the classroom is transformed into a 'pretend' hospital, so as to familiarise the children with some hospital procedures.

Resources

Action for Sick Children, Action for Sick Children's Schools Pack, 1998

Carter, M., *You and Your Child in Hospital*, Methuen, 1989

Claxton, R. and Harrison, T., *Caring for Children with HIV and AIDS*, Edward Arnold, 1991

Darbyshire, P., *Living with a Sick Child in Hospital*, Chapman Hall, 1994

Department of Health, *The Welfare of Young Children in Hospital*, HMSO, 1991

Gilbert, P., *The A-Z Reference Book of Syndromes and Inherited Diseases*, Stanley Thornes, 1996

  The A-Z Reference Book of Childhood Conditions, Chapman Hall, 1995

Harvey, S. and Hales Took, A. (Eds), *Play in Hospital*, Faber, 1979

Jolly, H., *The Other Side of Paediatrics*, MacMillan, 1981

Keene, A., *Care of the Child in Health and Sickness*, Stanley Thornes, 1999

Kubler Ross, E., *On Death and Dying*, Tavistock Publications, 1969

Lansdown, R., *Children in Hospital*, OUP, 1996

Lindsey, B. and Elsegood, J., *Working with Children in Grief and Loss*, Ballière Tindall, 1996

Valma, B., *The BMA Children's Symptoms*, Dorling Kindersley, 1997

Weller, B., *Helping Sick Children Play*, Balliere Tindall, 1980

Addresses

Action for Sick Children, Argyle House, London NW1 2SD. Telephone 0171 833 2041

Association for Children with Life Threatening and Terminal Illness, 65 St Michael's Road, Bristol BS2 8DZ. Telephone: 0117 922 1556

Cruse Bereavement Care, Cruse House, 126 Sheen Road, Richmond, Surrey TW9 1UR. Telephone: 0181 940 4818

Enuresis Resource and Information Centre, 65 St. Michael's Hill, Bristol BS2 8DZ. Telephone: 0117 926 4920

National Association of Hospital Play Staff, 40 Brunswick Square, London WC1N 1AZ. Telephone: 0171 278 2424

National Asthma Campaign, Providence House, Providence Place, London N1 0NT. Website: www.asthma.org.UK

National Eczema Society, 163 Eversholt Street, London NW1 1BU. Website: www.eczema.org.UK

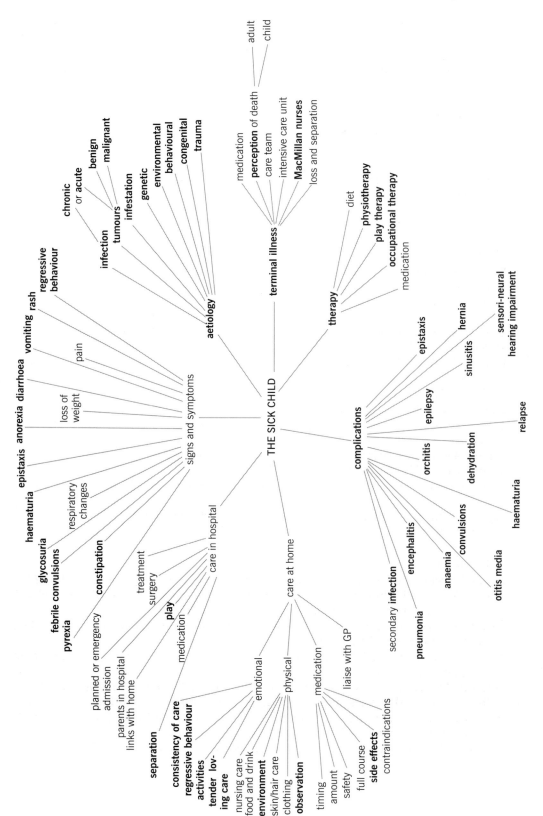

THE SICK CHILD

signs and symptoms
- vomiting
- rash
- regressive behaviour
- diarrhoea
- anorexia
- epistaxis
- haematuria
- glycosuria
- febrile convulsions
- pyrexia
- constipation
- respiratory changes
- loss of weight
- pain

aetiology
- infection
- tumours
  - chronic or acute
  - benign
  - malignant
- infestation
- genetic
- environmental
- behavioural
- congenital
- trauma

terminal illness
- medication
- perception of death
  - adult
  - child
- care team
- intensive care unit
- MacMillan nurses
- loss and separation

therapy
- diet
- physiotherapy
- play therapy
- occupational therapy
- medication

complications
- epistaxis
- hernia
- sinusitis
- sensori-neural hearing impairment
- epilepsy
- orchitis
- dehydration
- relapse
- encephalitis
- convulsions
- anaemia
- haematuria
- secondary infection
- pneumonia
- otitis media

care in hospital
- treatment
- surgery
- play
- medication
- planned or emergency admission
- parents in hospital
- links with home
- separation
- consistency of care
- regressive behaviour
- activities
- tender loving care

care at home
- emotional
- physical
- medication
- liaise with GP
- nursing care
- food and drink
- environment
- skin/hair care
- clothing
- observation
- timing
- amount
- safety
- full course
- side effects
- contraindications

23 *Children and society*

Society is always changing and so are child-rearing practices. You need to be aware of all the legislation concerning children, and the impact of social changes on children.

You will need to read quality newspapers to keep up to date with social trends and policies. You may find yourself lobbying MPs or joining pressure groups so as to protect disadvantaged children.

Resources

Allen, N., *Making Sense of the Children Act, 1989*, Longman, 1990
Bradshaw, J., *Child Poverty and Deprivation in the UK*, NCB, 1990
Department of Health, *The Rights of the Child*, HMSO, 1993
Dewar, J., *Law and the Family*, Butterworth, 1992
Hill, M., *Understanding Social Policy* (4th edn), Blackwell, 1993
Kumar, V., *Poverty and Inequality in the UK*, NCB, 1993
Leach, P., *Children First*, Michael Joseph, 1994
Miller, J., *Never Too Young*, National Early Years Network, 1997
Newell, P., *The UN Convention and Children's Rights in the UK*, NCB, 1991
Pugh, G. (Ed), *Contemporary Issues in the Early Years*, Paul Chapman, 1992
Triseliotis, J. et al, *Adoption*, Cassell, 1997
Webb, R. and Tossell, D., *Social Issues for Carers*, Edward Arnold, 1991
Wyld, N., *Responsibility for Under Eights: a guide to the law*, National Early Years Network, 1996

Addresses

British Agencies for Adoption and Fostering, 11 Southwark Street, London SE1 1RQ. Website: www.vois.org.UK/baaf/
Child Poverty Action Group (CPAG), 1–5 Bath Street, London EC1V 9PY. Telephone: 0171 253 3406. Website: staff@cpag.demon.co.UK
Children's Legal Centre, University of Essex, Wivenhoe Park, Colchester, Essex CO4 3SQ. Telephone: 01206 873 820
Children's Rights Office, 235 Shaftesbury Avenue, London WC2H 8EL. Telephone: 0171 278 8222
Department for Education and Employment, Sanctuary Buildings, Great Smith Street, London SW1P 3BT
Family Welfare Association, 501 Kingsland Road, Hackney, London E8 4AU. Telephone: 0171 254 6251
Grandparents Federation, Moot House, The Stow, Harlow, Essex CH20 3AG
National Council for One Parent Families, 255 Kentish Town Road, London NW5 2LX. Telephone: 0171 267 1361
National Step-family Association, Chapel House, 18 Hatton Place, London EC1N 8JH. Telephone: 0171 209 2460. Website: www.webcreations.co.UK/national.step-family
Office for Standards in Education (OFSTED), Alexandra House, 33 Kingsway, London WC1B 6SE
Shelter, 88 Old Street, London EC1V 9HU. Telephone: 0171 253 0202. Website: www.shelter.org.UK

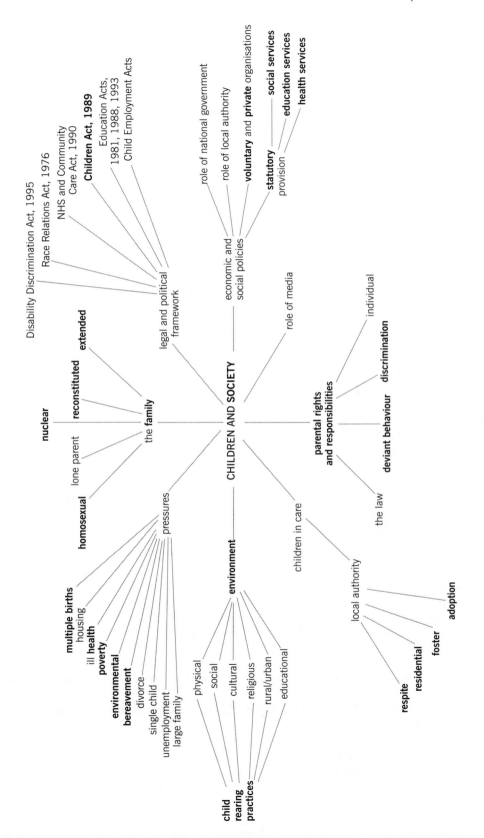

24 Children with disabilities

The term 'disabilities' is used to describe those children whose development may be delayed due to a physical, emotional, language or cognitive impairment.

You will find children with disabilities in mainstream schools and nurseries, sometimes supported by individual carers, or within special schools and units. They have exactly the same needs as other children and it is important not to label them, or allow their disability to distort the way you care for them. After just a few days of contact, you will learn to see the child and not the disability. A sound understanding of child development will allow you to plan and prepare activities to encourage their development and education.

Resources

ACE Special Education Handbook, *The Law on Children with Special Needs*, ACE, 1996

Dare, A. and O'Donovan, M., *Good Practice in Caring for Young Children with Special Needs*, Stanley Thornes, 1997

Fox, G., *A Handbook for Special Needs Assistants*, David Fulton, 1993

Hall, D., *Health for All Children*, OUP, 1996

PLA, *Play and Learning for All Children: children with special needs in playgroups*, PLA, 1993

Rieser, R. and Mason, M., *Disability in the Classroom: Human Rights*, Disability Equality in Education, 1992

Sherborne, V., *Developmental Movement for Children*, CUP, 1996

Woolfson, J., *Children with Special Needs*, Faber and Faber, 1991

Addresses

Association for Spina Bifida and Hydrocephalus (ASBAH), 42 Park Road, Peterborough PE1 2UQ. Website: www.asbah.demon.co.UK

British Deaf Association, 1–3 Worship Street, London EC2 2AB. Website: www.bda.org.UK

Contact a Family, 170 Tottenham Court Road, London W1P 0HA

Council for Disabled Children, 8 Wakely Street, London EC1V 7QE

Disabled Living Foundation, 380–384 Harrow Road, London W9 2HU

Down's Syndrome Educational Trust. Website: www.downsnet.org

HAPA, Pryor's Bank, Bishop's Park, London SW6 3AL. Telephone: 0171 731 1435

MIND (National Association for Mental Health), Granta House, Broadway, London E15. Telephone: 0181 519 2122. Website: www.mind.org.UK

Muscular Dystrophy Group, Nattrass House, 35 Macaulay Road, London SW4 0QP. Website: www.sonnet.co.UK/muscular-dystrophy.html

The National Association for Special Educational Needs, Nasen House, 4–5 Amber Business Village, Amber Close, Amington, Tamworth B77 4RP

Royal National Institute for the Blind, 224 Great Portland Street, London W1N 6AA. Website: www.rnib.org.UK

SCOPE (Cerebral Palsy Society), London and SE Regional Office, Shackleton Square, Priestley Way, Crawley. Telephone: 01293 522 655 (helpline 0800 626 216). Website: www.nspcc.org.UK

SENSE (The National Deaf, Blind and Rubella Association), 11–13 Clifton Terrace, Finsbury Park, London N4 3SR

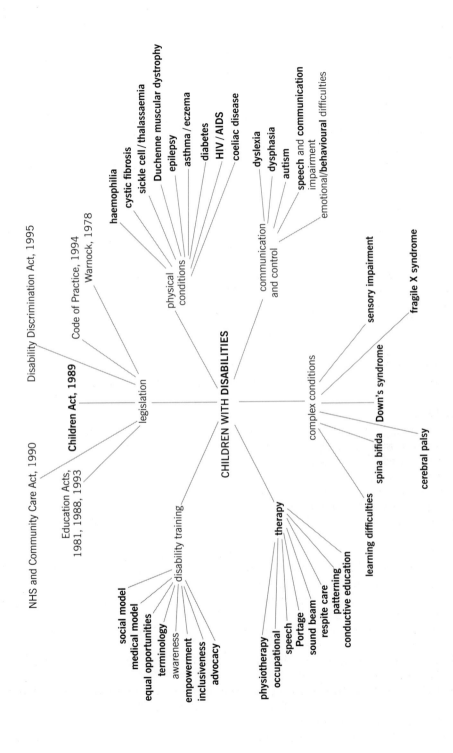

CHILDREN WITH DISABILITIES

legislation
- NHS and Community Care Act, 1990
- Education Acts, 1981, 1988, 1993
- Disability Discrimination Act, 1995
- **Children Act, 1989**
- Code of Practice, 1994
- Warnock, 1978

physical conditions
- haemophilia
- **cystic fibrosis**
- sickle cell / thalassaemia
- **Duchenne muscular dystrophy**
- epilepsy
- asthma / eczema
- diabetes
- **HIV / AIDS**
- coeliac disease

communication and control
- dyslexia
- dysphasia
- autism
- **speech** and **communication** impairment
- emotional/**behavioural** difficulties

complex conditions
- sensory impairment
- **fragile X syndrome**
- **Down's syndrome**
- spina bifida
- cerebral palsy
- learning difficulties

disability training
- social model
- medical model
- equal opportunities
- terminology
- awareness
- **empowerment**
- **inclusiveness**
- advocacy

therapy
- physiotherapy
- occupational
- speech
- **Portage**
- **sound beam**
- respite care
- patterning
- **conductive education**

25 Employment

There are many areas of employment for people with a childcare qualification. The traditional role of parents has changed during the last twenty-five years, resulting in a demand for more childcare provision. Other changes in society have led to new employment opportunities, such as working alongside health professionals. There are now many settings and structures within which you can seek employment.

When considering your future career, it is necessary that you understand the importance of job search, application and interview. You should obtain a job description and a contract outlining your conditions of service. When in employment, you need to demonstrate awareness of good professional practice, knowledge of different management styles, employment protection acts, and policies and procedures.

Resources

Clark, A., 'What do Nursery Nurses do?' in *Nursery World*, 2.6.94
Cowley, L., et al, *Young Children in Group Daycare: guidelines for good practice*, National Children's Bureau, 1991
Hobart, C. and Frankel, J., *A Practical Guide To Childcare Employment*, Stanley Thornes, 1996
Sadek, E. and Sadek, J., *Good Practice in Nursery Management*, Stanley Thornes, 1996
Taylor, G., *Equal Opportunities*, The Industrial Society, 1994

Addresses

Council for Awards in Children's Care and Education (CACHE), 8 Chequer Street, St Albans, Herts AL1 2XZ. Telephone: 01727 847 636 or 01727 867333. Website: http://ourworld.compuserve.com/homepages/CACHE
The Federation of Recruitment and Employment Services (FRES), 36 Mortimer Street, London W1N 7RB. Telephone: 0171 323 4300
The Industrial Society, Peter Runge House, 3 Carlton House Terrace, London SW1Y 2DG. Telephone: 0171 839 4300
National Association of Nursery Nurses (NANN), 17 Lamb Close, Garston, Watford, Herts WD2 6TB. Telephone: 01923 893967
Professional Association of Nursery Nurses (PANN), 2 St James's Court, Friar Gate, Derby DE1 1BT. Telephone: 01332 343029
The Public Service Union (UNISON), Unison Centre, Holborn Tower, 137 High Holborn, London WC1V 6PL. Telephone: 0171 388 2366

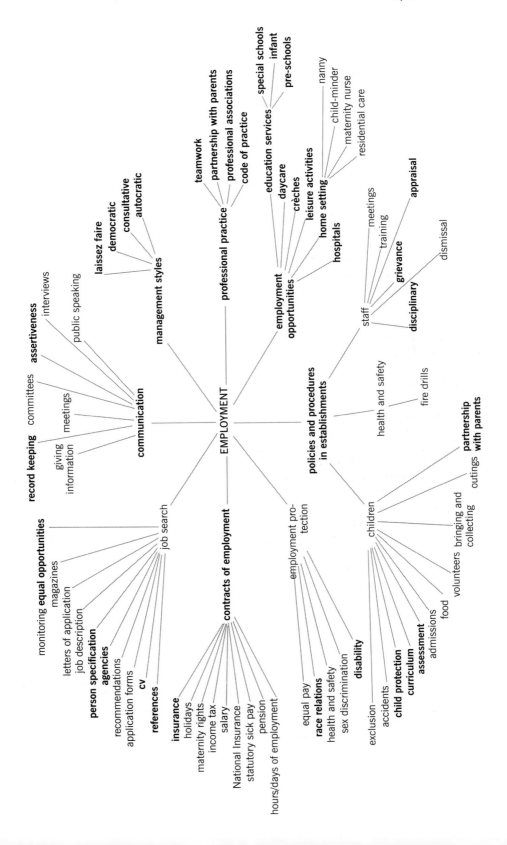

EMPLOYMENT

communication
- **record keeping**
- committees
- **assertiveness**
- interviews
- public speaking
- giving information
- meetings

management styles
- laissez faire
- democratic
- **consultative**
- autocratic

professional practice
- **teamwork**
- **partnership with parents**
- **professional associations**
- **code of practice**

employment opportunities
- **education services**
  - special schools
  - infant
  - **pre-schools**
- daycare
- **crèches**
- **leisure activities**
- **home setting**
  - nanny
  - child-minder
  - maternity nurse
  - residential care
- **hospitals**

staff
- meetings
- training
- **appraisal**
- **grievance**
- **disciplinary**
- dismissal

policies and procedures in establishments
- health and safety
- fire drills

children
- **partnership with parents**
- bringing and collecting
- outings
- volunteers
- food
- admissions
- **assessment**
- **curriculum**
- **child protection**
- accidents
- exclusion
- **disability**
- sex discrimination
- health and safety
- **race relations**
- equal pay

contracts of employment
- employment protection
- hours/days of employment
- pension
- statutory sick pay
- National Insurance
- salary
- income tax
- maternity rights
- holidays
- **insurance**

job search
- **references**
- **cv**
- application forms
- recommendations
- **agencies**
- **person specification**
- job description
- letters of application
- magazines
- monitoring **equal opportunities**

26 Maintaining good health in children

To make sure that the children in your care are healthy, you will be working in partnership with their parents. A childcare practitioner is a health educator who wishes to promote the health of children by understanding health issues and being a good role model.

You will understand the importance of routine surveillance and screening programmes, and encourage parents to participate.

Resources

Audit Commission, *Seen But Not Heard: co-ordinating community child health and social services for children in need*, HMSO, 1994

Bax, M. et al, *Child Development and Child Health*, Blackwell Scientific, 1990

Brown, H. (Ed.), *Which Guide to Child Health*, Which Books, 1997

Department of Health, *Child Health in the Community*, HMSO, 1996; and *Services for children and young people*. Telephone the Health Literature Line: 0800 555 777 for a free copy

   The Children Act, 1989: an introductory guide for the NHS, HMSO, 1991

Edwards, M., *Medical Symptoms in Children*, Foulsham, 1994

Elfer, P. and Gatiss, S., *Charting Child Health Services*, NCB, 1990

Hall, D. (Ed.), *Health for all Children*, Oxford Medical Publishers, 1989

Hall, D. et al, *The Child Surveillance Handbook* (2nd edn), Radcliffe Medical Press, 1994

Hollyer, B. and Smith, L., *Sleep: the secret of problem free nights*, Ward Lock, 1996

   Feeding: the simple solution, Ward Lock, 1997

Illingworth, R., *The Development of the Infant and the Young Child* (9th edn), Churchill Livingstone, 1987

Jolly, H., *Book of Child Care*, Unwin, 1985

Keene, A., *Care of the Child in Health and Sickness*, Stanley Thornes, 1999

Kurtz, Z. and Bahl, V. (Eds), *The Health and Health Care of Children and Young People from Minority Ethnic Groups in Britain*, NCB and Dept of Health, 1997

Minett, P. et al, *Human Form and Function*, Unwin Hyman, 1989

Moreton, J. and Macfarlane, A., *Child Health and Surveillance* (2nd edn), Blackwell Scientific Publishers, 1991

Naidoo, J. and Wills, J., *Health Promotion*, Ballière Tindall, 1994

Nash, W. et al, *Health at School*, Butterworth Heinemann, 1985

Pollak, M., *Textbook of Developmental Paediatrics*, Churchill Livingstone, 1993

Spencer, N. (Ed.), *Progress in Community Child Health*, Churchill Livingstone, 1998

Valman, H., *ABC of 1–7 years* (2nd edn), BMJ, 1993

Volcuf (now Early Years Network), *Keeping Children Healthy*, 1991

Addresses

Department of Health, Richmond House, 79 Whitehall, London SW1A 2NS. Telephone: 0171 210 4850 **also** Wellington House, 133–155 Waterloo Road, London, SE1 8UG. Telephone: 0171 972 2000

American Medical Association, Children's Health. Website: http://www.ama-assn.org

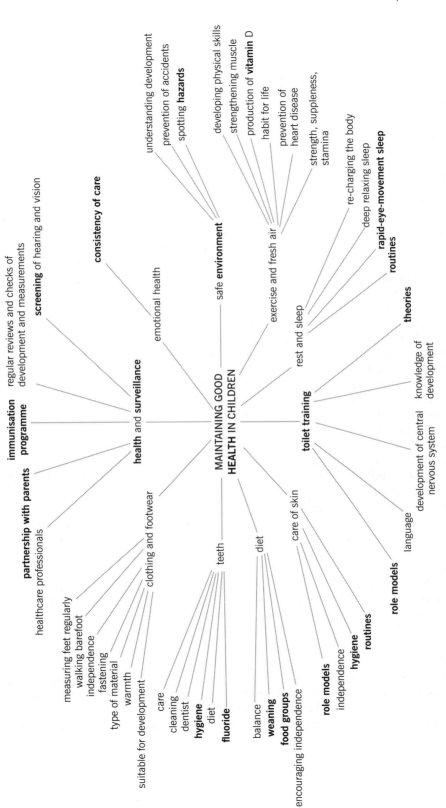

MAINTAINING GOOD HEALTH IN CHILDREN

health and surveillance
- regular reviews and checks of development and measurements
- screening of hearing and vision
- consistency of care
- immunisation programme
- partnership with parents
  - healthcare professionals
- emotional health

safe environment
- understanding development
- prevention of accidents
- spotting hazards

exercise and fresh air
- developing physical skills
- strengthening muscle
- production of vitamin D
- habit for life
- prevention of heart disease
- strength, suppleness, stamina

rest and sleep
- re-charging the body
- deep relaxing sleep
- rapid-eye-movement sleep
- routines

toilet training
- theories
- knowledge of development
- development of central nervous system
- language
- role models
- hygiene
- routines
- independence
- encouraging independence

care of skin
- role models
- hygiene
- routines

diet
- balance
- weaning
- food groups

teeth
- clothing and footwear
- care
- cleaning
- dentist
- hygiene
- diet
- fluoride

clothing and footwear
- measuring feet regularly
- walking barefoot
- independence
- fastening
- type of material
- warmth
- suitable for development

27 *Playwork*

Playwork refers to a range of settings providing play opportunities for children out of school, without their parents being present. These play opportunities could be after-school clubs and playschemes, holiday schemes or adventure playgrounds.

The provision is mainly for children five years and older. The government is committed to investing resources in after-school clubs to enable parents to return to work. There are recognised National Vocational Qualifications (NVQs) for people wishing to work in these settings.

Resources

Bonel, P., *Playing for Real*, Children's Play and Recreation, 1993
Bonel, P. and Lindon, J., *Good Practice in Playwork*, Stanley Thornes, 1996
Kids' Clubs Network, *Guidelines of Good Practice for Out of School Care Schemes*, 1993
Lubelska, A., *Key Issues in Play*, NCB, 1997
Petrie, P., *Play and care, out of School*, HMSO, 1994

Addresses

Kids' Clubs Network, Bellerive House, 3 Muirfield Crescent, London E14 G52
Joint National Committee of Training for Playwork, The Three Mills Play and Training Centre, 1 Abbey Lane, Stratford, London E15 2SD. Telephone: 0181 519 1908
National Play Information Centre and National Voluntary Council for Children's Play, 359–361 Euston Road, London NW1 3AL
Real Play Network, 14 Glebe Road, Reading, Berks RG2 7AG

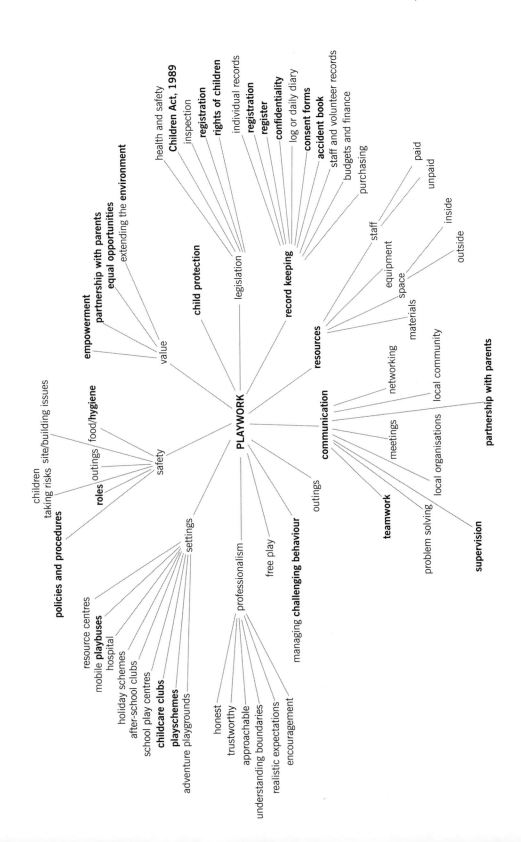

PLAYWORK

empowerment
partnership with parents
equal opportunities
extending the **environment**

health and safety
Children Act, 1989
inspection
registration
rights of children
individual records
registration
register
confidentiality
log or daily diary
consent forms
accident book
staff and volunteer records
budgets and finance
purchasing

child protection

legislation

value

record keeping

paid
unpaid

staff

equipment
space
inside
materials
outside

resources

children
taking risks   site/building issues

policies and procedures

roles   outings   **food/hygiene**

safety

communication

networking

meetings

local community

local organisations

outings

problem solving

teamwork

partnership with parents

supervision

resource centres
mobile **playbuses**
hospital
holiday schemes
after-school clubs
school play centres
childcare clubs
playschemes
adventure playgrounds

settings

professionalism

free play

managing **challenging behaviour**

honest
trustworthy
approachable
understanding boundaries
realistic expectations
encouragement

PART THREE: CHILDCARE DICTIONARY

This section of the book consists of a dictionary of around 1,000 key terms that you may encounter in your course, including theorists and, at the end of the dictionary, all those confusing acronyms and abbreviations you come across!

Each term is clearly defined and, where another dictionary term is referred to within a definition, that term appears in italics. In this way, and through the links with the topic webs in the previous section, you can quickly and easily develop an understanding of all the key areas and issues you are likely to encounter in your childcare course.

Dictionary

A

ableism
Discrimination in favour of able-bodied people.

abortion
An interruption or termination of pregnancy before the *fetus* is *viable* and capable of living outside the *uterus*. It can be a spontaneous abortion (*miscarriage*), occurring by itself, or induced and deliberately caused by human action.

abrasion
A wound where the skin is scraped or worn away with little or no damage to underlying tissues (sometimes referred to as a 'graze').

abscess
A cavity containing pus resulting from *infection* by *bacteria*.

absences (petit mal)
A milder type of epileptic fit. The child looks vacant and pale, the head may droop. It lasts only a few seconds but the child is completely cut off from his or her surroundings. See *epilepsy*.

abuse
See *child protection*.

accents
The way that people pronounce words and sounds are unique to them. Sometimes the accent is shared in some way with other people, and is categorised as, for example, 'cockney' or 'French'.

accident book
A health and safety requirement in all establishments for accurate recording of who was involved, what occurred, details of any injury and treatment, and who was informed of the accident.

accommodation
In *Piaget*'s terminology, describes changes in existing *cognitive* structures to include new experiences.

achondroplasia
Associated with short but strong arms and legs with a short body and a slightly protruding forehead.

acquired immune deficiency syndrome (AIDS)
Caused by a *virus* and transmitted through body fluids. The body loses its ability to resist *infection*. The lymph nodes enlarge and often a *cancer* that affects the skin develops. The virus is very delicate and dies quickly outside the body.

active immunity
Acquired by the body either suffering an illness and responding by producing *antibodies* or *antitoxins*; **or** by *immunisation* with a weakened form of the *bacteria* so that the body forms antibodies or antitoxins without having to suffer the actual illness.

activities with children
The *pre-school curriculum* that should always be well planned and prepared, taking into account the *areas of development* that the particular activity will promote and extend.

acute conditions
An illness that comes on suddenly and is of short-term duration.

adaptation
According to *Piaget*, this is the term used to describe the complementary procedures of *accommodation* and *assimilation* resulting in a change in *behaviour*.

admiral nurses
Trained nurses who specialise in looking after dementia patients in their own homes, and in supporting their relatives/carers.

adoption
To care legally for another's child as one's own child with full *parental responsibility*.

adrenaline
A *hormone* secreted in response to stress that increases heart and pulse rates and blood pressure.

adult interaction
The adult will *play* and interact with the child, or children, extending learning and language.

adult intervention
The adult will intervene in the *play*, often preventing the children from *creative* and *imaginative play*. Intervention might be necessary if the play becomes dangerous, or if it becomes too *repetitive*.

advocacy
Active support of a cause or argument. Interceding on behalf of another person.

aesthetic development
Aestheticism takes time to develop, and can be helped by a stimulating and beautiful *environment*, the appreciation of which leads to an understanding of the man-made and the natural world. As the appreciation of the aesthetic develops, there will be a response of the *senses*, an understanding of patterns, an ability to select materials, and an enjoyment of *displayed* work, including museums and art galleries.

aetiology
The cause of a disease.

affective disorder
An emotional disorder. A child, who is emotionally disturbed, may display *behaviour* that is *aggressive*, *regressive*, *withdrawn* or *antisocial*.

agency
A business or organisation with a specific *role* and function.

aggressive behaviour
This describes *behaviour* that is disruptive, verbally *aggressive*, physically aggressive, defiant, resorting to *tantrums*, and disobedience.

albino
A person of any *race* who has a *congenital* absence of the pigment melanin in the skin, hair, and eyes. The pink eyes are a reflection of the blood vessels through the tissues.

allergen
Any substance, such as food, fur, pollen, and dust, that is usually harmless, but provokes an allergic reaction in susceptible individuals.

allergy
An *acute* reaction of the body to something eaten, inhaled or touched (an *allergen*), to which previous exposure has made the body sensitive. It is a misdirected response by the body involving the production of *antibodies* against otherwise harmless substances.

alopecia
Bald patches or total loss of hair.

amino acids
The chemical structure of *proteins*. Digestion breaks down the protein into amino acids and it is then built up again into the type of protein required by the body such as muscle fibres, plasma proteins, *enzymes*, and collagen fibre in bone and cartilage.

amnesia
Complete or partial loss of memory.

amniocentesis
Antenatal procedure carried out at 16–18 weeks. A fine needle is inserted into the *uterus* and a sample of amniotic fluid is withdrawn. This can be tested for *Down's syndrome*, *spina bifida* and *muscular dystrophy*. The results of the test are usually known in about three weeks.

anaemia
A blood disorder in which there is a *deficiency* of red blood cells, haemoglobin, or both. Poor diet, loss of blood or bone marrow disease are among the causes.

anal fissures
Hard *stools* can tear the lining membrane inside the anus, producing a fissure (crack). May be an indicator of *sexual abuse*.

anal stage
Freud's term for the psychosexual stage in which a young child finds gratification through the body and bodily products. Poor toilet training can lead to a fixation at this stage together with a reluctance to excrete faeces, leading to constipation. In adult life, a person who is inflexible and controlling is sometimes called 'anal-retentive'.

analgesics
A group of drugs that relieve pain.

anaphylaxis
A generalised *allergic* reaction. It can result in a total collapse of the body.

anatomy
The science of the structure of the body of animals describing the form and arrangement of the parts of the body.

androgynous
Having male and female characteristics.

anorexia
Loss of appetite.

anorexia nervosa
An eating disorder, where the sufferer has a distorted image of his or her own body shape.

anosmia
Loss of sense of smell.

anoxia
Lack or deficiency of oxygen in body tissues. Lack of oxygen to the brain will cause brain damage.

antenatal
Before birth.

anthropomorphism
The attribution of human form or *behaviour* to other animals.

antibiotics
Drugs that kill *bacteria* or stop their growth.

antibodies
Complex substances formed to neutralise or destroy *antigens*. Their activity fights *infection*.

anti-discriminatory practice
Examining all areas of practice to ensure that no *discrimination* occurs, that all resources project *positive images* and that the language used, including *naming systems*, is appropriate and correct, and that all *prejudice* and discrimination is challenged. All childcare practitioners must be aware of *equal opportunity* policies, and implement them in their workplace.

anti-emetics
Drugs to prevent *vomiting*.

antigen
Any foreign substance, such as *micro-organisms* and *vaccines* that can be detected by the body's *immune system*. Detection stimulates the formation of *antibodies*.

antihistamine
Drugs taken to prevent or reduce an *allergic* reaction.

antiseptic
A solution that prevents or stops the growth of *pathogenic micro-organisms*. It may be applied to the skin but is too powerful to be swallowed or injected into the body.

antisocial behaviour
Unacceptable *behaviour*, resulting in pain, destruction of property and emotional distress.

antitoxin
A substance that neutralises the effects of a *toxin*.

apathetic
Having or showing little emotion or interest.

Apgar scale
Used to measure the condition of the *newborn*, assessing muscle tone, pulse, colour, response to stimulus and respiration. Each area is given a score from nought to two, with a maximum total of ten. The test is applied when the baby is one minute old and repeated at five-minute intervals until the score of ten is achieved.

aphagia
Loss of the power to swallow.

aphasia
Loss of the power of speech or of understanding the written or spoken word.

aphonia
Inability to produce vocal sound.

appraisal
A term used to describe the procedure of assessing staff on their work and practice on a regular basis. This helps them to look at their progress and self-development, and decide what further training might help them and the establishment in the future.

areas of development
When caring for children, it is necessary to be aware of their total development, which includes *physical, cognitive, language, social, emotional, moral, spiritual, creative* and *aesthetic* development.

arthritis
Inflammation of the joints and the surrounding tissues.

artificial immunity
Includes *vaccination* where the body is given a weakened form of the *micro-organism* to stimulate the

production of *antibodies* or a *serum* obtained from another person or animal that contains antibodies.

aseptic
Free of *pathogens*.

asphyxia
Failure to breathe.

assertiveness
A way of dealing with threatening or difficult situations in a firm but non-*aggressive* way. Assertiveness training is available on some childcare courses.

assessment
Children may be assessed in many different ways using various techniques. Reports may be written for parents, records (see *record keeping*) are kept at the school, physical prowess is recorded and social *behaviour* is noted. It is important to assess children frequently, so that one has an objective view of their ability, and can plan to promote and extend their *areas of development*.

assimilation
In *Piaget*'s terminology, the term used to describe the incorporation of a new experience, object, or *concept* into existing *cognitive* structures.

associative play
Playing in a group of children.

assumption
Accepting that something is true, without any evidence.

asthma
A lung condition where the airway is obstructed due to muscle spasm and the secretion of excessive amounts of *mucus*; it may result from *allergy*, emotional factors or *infection*.

astigmatism
The lens of the eye is not smooth, objects will look crooked or out of shape.

asymmetrical movements
Jerky, uncoordinated movements of the body.

ataxia
Lack of co-ordination in body movement due to some form of nerve or brain damage.

athetosis
An involuntary sinuous writhing movement seen in some children with *cerebral palsy*.

atresia
Congenital blockage of a body orifice, for example the anus, or complete absence of a passageway, such as the oesophagus (the gullet). It is life threatening but can be treated with surgery.

attachment
Feeling affection, even devotion, for another, which is always reciprocated, often between parent and child.

attention deficit hyperactivity disorder (ADHD)
A behaviour disorder that causes disruption in the classroom, as the child appears unable to keep still and attend. Sometimes treated, controversially, with drugs, usually Ritalin. Food additives and emotional problems have been seen as possible causes of the disorder.

attention seeking
Inappropriate behaviour, demanding attention, often by disruptive behaviour.

au pair
A young person who goes to another country mainly to learn the language. Usually, au pairs like to work with children, but being untrained and inexperienced, they should be supervised, live as part of the family, and given plenty of time to study and be with friends.

audiology
The study of hearing, often including the diagnosis and treatment of people with hearing defects.

auditory
Relating to hearing.

auditory discrimination
The ability to hear and tell the difference between different sounds and frequencies. Good auditory discrimination aids *language development*.

autism
A disorder of normal *cognitive* function and *language development* and describes a condition that makes it difficult for people to *communicate* adequately with others, therefore resulting in problems in making relationships. Autistic people often show complete self-absorption, and many have obsessional habits. Some autistic children are gifted in music, mathematics and/or drawing. Infantile autism begins in the first few months of life and is also known as *Kanner's syndrome*. Research has recently shown that

autism may be inherited, as a *gene* has been identified which shows a predisposition to autism.

autocratic
See *management styles*.

automatic nervous system
Involuntary responses that regulate many body activities such as digestion or response to stress.

axilla
The armpit.

B

babbling
Pre-linguistic speech, in which infants repeat certain sounds.

bacteria
Single cell *micro-organisms*, which can only be seen under the microscope. Not all cause disease. They are divided into groups determined by their shape, cocci (round), bacilli (rod-shaped), and vibrios (curved). They reproduce themselves at a very rapid rate to damage body tissues, and can produce poisons (*toxins*) which cause more damage.

bar charts
A way of showing collected *data* in a graphic fashion, with each chunk of data in a column.

barrier nursing
To care for patients who are infectious or who have poor *immunity*, in *isolation* to prevent the spread of *infection*.

battered child syndrome
A term first coined in 1962 to describe *physical abuse* of a child.

BCG vaccine
An injection against TB (*tuberculosis*).

behaviour
Total response, an individual's actions and reactions.

behaviour modification
To change *behaviour* successfully, it is necessary for all the adults working with the child to work together with consistent guidelines, giving plenty of attention, and rewarding 'good' behaviour, while ignoring 'bad' behaviour. It uses the principles of *behaviourism* to alter behaviour.

behaviourism
The study of observable *behaviours* and events, which emphasises the role of the *environment* in causing behaviour.

bell curve
In statistics, most commonly used when testing a person's *intelligence quotient*, the shape of a bell is used to show that most people fall in the middle or median, with just a few who have a much higher or much lower intelligence.

benign
Showing kindness; **or** may refer to a *tumour* that is non-*malignant*, harmless or curable.

bereavement
Grieving for the loss of a person or an animal who has died. The classic symptoms are shock, denial, searching, guilt, anger and fear.

bias
Showing a preference or predisposition towards individuals, groups or ideas.

bibliography
The listing of books read and used in an essay, a book or a piece of research.

bilingualism
The ability to speak two languages fluently. A term often used in schools to describe children who speak one language at home (*heritage language*) and another in school.

biopsy
Removal of a small piece of tissue from the body for microscopic analysis.

birth order
The birth of a child within a family in relation to any *siblings*.

birth-rate
The ratio of live births expressed per thousand population per year.

bisexuality
Emotional and sexual relationships with people of either *gender*.

body language
See *non-verbal communication*.

boils
Abscesses in the skin caused by *staphylococcal bacteria*.

bonding
Becoming emotionally attached to one person, and usually describes the *attachment* of the mother to the *newborn*, and of the newborn to the mother.

bottle-feeding
The practice of offering fluids to a baby in a bottle, it may contain water, expressed breast milk or *formula milk*.

botulism
Rare food poisoning caused by *bacteria* found in faulty canned or preserved foods.

Bowlby, John (1907–1990)
British *ethological* theorist who worked at the Tavistock clinic and for the World Health Organisation. In 1951, in a paper given at the World Health Organisation, quoting a small retrospective study of 36 juvenile thieves, he pronounced that it was the deprivation of maternal attention that led to crime. He was influential in making mothers feel guilty if they went to work, arguing that they needed to be present during children's formative years in order for *bonding* to take place.

Braille
The alphabet used by severely visually impaired people, consisting of raised dots that have a different pattern for each letter, that enables them to read.

breast-feeding
The natural way of feeding a baby with milk produced by the mother and specific to each individual baby. It adapts to match the baby's *growth* and needs.

British Sign Language
A particular way of signing words with the hands, taught in many schools for the partially hearing.

bronchitis
An inflammation of the bronchi, the tubes leading from the windpipe (trachea) to the lung tissue (alveoli). It usually results from a viral upper respiratory tract *infection*.

Bruner, Jerome (1915–)
American psychologist. Influenced the *curriculum*. Eminent in this country for the Oxford *pre-school* research group. Pioneered techniques for investigating infant *perception*.

bulimia nervosa
An eating disorder of compulsive over-eating followed by *vomiting*.

bullying
Attacks on a child, which can be physical, emotional, verbal, racist and/or sexual. In its extreme form it can lead to suicide in young people and is the main cause of school refusal. It can leave emotional scars that remain for life.

C

Caesarean section
An operation under general or *epidural anaesthesia* where the baby is delivered through a cut in the abdominal wall.

calcium
A mineral found in *dairy foods*, pulses, fish and green vegetables. It is essential for growth and maintenance of strong bones and teeth. Lack of calcium in the diet leads to caries, rickets, muscle cramps and delayed blood clotting.

calorie
A unit of energy.

cancer
A disorder of cell growth.

capacity and volume
Volume is the amount of space taken up by an object. Capacity is the amount an object can contain.

carbohydrate
One of the main food groups, essential for warmth and energy, it can be divided into sugars and starches. Sugars convert quickly to glucose and are a fast source of energy. Starches take longer to convert and provide a longer lasting source of energy.

carbohydrate foods
Starchy *carbohydrates*, such as bread, cereals and pasta are essential to the diet as they also provide other essential nutrients.

caries
Dental decay, which may be prevented by a good diet, avoiding sugar, regular teeth brushing, regular dental checks and *fluoride*.

carrier
A person whose body carries *pathogenic organisms* without developing the symptoms of the disease, who can pass the *infection* on to others: **or** a person who

carries a *gene* for a hereditary disorder that may be passed on to his or her children.

case history
A record of an individual's background, health status, education, and life experience.

case study
An example of a particular situation to illustrate a theoretical point.

catarrh
The profuse nasal discharge that accompanies a cold.

central nervous system
The brain and spinal cord.

central register
The name of the child protection register on which the names of children at risk are placed.

cephalhaematoma
A blood-filled swelling on the baby's head caused by the rupture of small blood vessels during labour.

cerebral palsy
Occurs as a result of damage to the developing brain, during pregnancy or at birth, affecting the areas that control movement.

cerebrospinal fluid
The clear liquid around the brain and spinal cord.

challenging behaviour
Describes the child displaying *behaviour* that is inappropriate and attention seeking. The causes of challenging behaviour may be due to many factors. Some are the results of normal development, such as a wish to be independent, frustration, *egocentricity*, or curiosity. Others may be due to *abuse*, *neglect* or poor parenting skills and can show in the child as anger, fear, or anxiety. Frustrated emotional needs and the need to seek attention cause most challenging behaviour.

check list
One way of recording observations. A list of attributes is drawn up and the *behaviour*, *physical growth* or *language development* of the child is checked against it. It is then easy to see if the child is mature or immature for his or her chronological age, so that programmes can be planned to extend and promote particular *areas of development*.

chicken pox
An infectious disease caused by the herpes zoster

virus. It mainly affects the skin and lining of the throat and mouth.

chilblains
Red, painful, itching swellings in the extremities of the body.

child abuse and neglect
The different categories are *sexual abuse*, *emotional abuse*, *physical abuse and injury*, *organised (ritual) abuse*, *failure to thrive*, *Munchausen's syndrome by proxy*, *emotional neglect*, *physical neglect*, and *educational neglect*.

child abuse indicators
To recognise abuse there may be *physical* signs, such as bruises or burn marks, and/or *behavioural* indicators, such as withdrawal from relationships and crying, or being the subject of *bullying*. *Disclosure* from the child to an understanding adult is often the first indicator of *sexual abuse*.

child abuse inquiries
Inquiries are usually made after there has been a death from *child abuse* or *neglect*. Often the inquiry will lead to changes being made to protect children. Inquiries may also take place following allegations of large-scale abuse, for example, of children in *residential care*.

child abuse, some main factors
There are many theories that try to explain why people abuse or neglect children: *domestic violence*, *social and environmental factors*, *predisposing factors*, and *psychological factors*.

child development
The scientific study of normal changes in children over time. These changes can be *physical*, *cognitive*, or *social and emotional*. They do not occur in isolation, each affects the others.

child guidance
Children with emotional, *behavioural* and school difficulties can be seen, with their *families* in a child guidance clinic or unit based in a child development centre. A *multi-disciplinary team* includes a child *psychiatrist*, *educational psychologist*, psychotherapist and psychiatric *social worker* and often a family therapist as well.

child prostitution
Children may be lured into sexual activity for payment for many reasons. Child prostitutes are often runaways from *abuse* or an unhappy home life, and

are preyed upon by pimps in return for food and shelter.

child protection

Protecting children from *abuse and neglect* is the duty of the whole community. There are many *statutory* and *voluntary agencies* involved, such as the law, the police, *social services*, the *health services*, the NSPCC, *ChildLine* and *education services*. Childcare practitioners are in the forefront of child protection, and are often the first to recognise the *indicators of abuse* and neglect.

child protection agencies

The agencies which have to protect children by law (*statutory*), are the *education services*, *health services*, *social services*, police, and the legal framework. The main voluntary agencies that exist to protect children are the NSPCC and *ChildLine*.

child protection conferences

Formal meetings are called when a child has *disclosed abuse*, or when signs and *indicators of abuse* are reported to one of the *child protection agencies*. One person from each of the *statutory* services will be present. If it is seen that there is cause for concern, a *child protection plan* will be drawn up to protect the child, and the child's name placed on the *central register*.

child protection plan

The plan devised at the *child protection conference* to protect the child.

child protection review

Children on the *central register* are reviewed at frequent intervals, to see if the situation has changed, and the child can be *deregistered*.

child rearing practices

Children are brought up in many different ways with, for example, some families believing in firm *discipline* for even the mildest infringement of the rules, while other parents have far fewer rules and allow the children a great deal of freedom. A good understanding of *cultural* and *class* influences is necessary for any person working with children.

child study

Longitudinal study of an individual child.

childcare clubs

Schemes being developed to help parents who work, and will add to the *extended day provision* already provided in some areas.

child-centred

The ideas for *play* come from the child, and so ensures the interest and motivation of the child or children concerned.

ChildLine

A telephone line set up to enable children to speak to a counsellor if they have been abused or neglected in any way, or fear that they are in danger.

childminder

A person, registered with the local authority as suitable, who looks after one to three children in his or her own home for payment.

Children Act, 1989

An act drawn up to resolve the conflicting areas of family privacy, professional power and the rights of children. The three main principles are: the welfare of the child is paramount; there should be as little delay as possible by the courts in deciding issues; and the court has to be satisfied that it is better to make an order than not to do so. It brings together the care and upbringing of children in both private and public law. This has had an impact on childcare provision with firm guidance on *registration* and inspection.

cholesterol

A fat-like substance found in the body and in animal products. A raised level in the body increases the risk of heart disease and *obesity*.

Chomsky, Noam (1928–)

American linguist and political activist. He stated that innate *cognitive* structures were built into the brain, that parts of the brain were there to understand language, that there was the ability to understand grammar, and that the physical mechanisms such as the tongue, lips and palette were already in place. He called this a 'language acquisition device' or LAD.

chorea

An involuntary irregular jerking movement.

chorionic villus sampling (CVS)

An *antenatal* procedure carried out around ten weeks. A small sample of tissue is taken from the *placenta* to test for *congenital disorders*.

chromosomes

Holders of the body's genetic material, found in the nuclei of each body cell.

chronic illness
Long-standing conditions, continuing over a period of time.

chronological age
The actual age of a person.

cilia
Short minute hairlike vibrating structures on the surface of some cells; **or** eyelashes.

circumcision
In the male child, it is the surgical removal of the foreskin, which covers the tip (glans) of the penis. Female circumcision is illegal in the UK, but is still carried out in many parts of Asia, Africa and the Middle East.

class
One way of categorising a society is to group people into different classes – upper, middle and working.

cleft palate
A vertical split along the midline of the *palate*, extending from behind the teeth to the cavity of the nose. Feeding is difficult. Surgery will be carried out during the first year of life. Associated with *hare lip*.

client/customer
A parent/carer who is purchasing care and education for a child; **or** 'clients' can be a term sometimes used by *social workers* to describe the families with whom they are involved.

code of practice
An ethical way of working defined by a professional body or establishment. A statement of values.

coeliac condition
A sensitivity to a *protein*, gluten, found in wheat and rye, damaging the wall of the small intestine, resulting in reduced ability to absorb nutrients. Results in a need for a gluten-free diet for life.

cognitive
Intellectual. Having the ability to understand and reason.

cognitive development
The development of the intellect, describing the changes in mental powers and qualities that permit understanding. It is thought that a person's intelligence is about 75 per cent due to inherited ability and the remaining 25 per cent to a loving and stimulating *environment*. *Piaget* states that it is the way

the one acts upon the other that develops cognitive ability.

colic
An intense, acute abdominal pain, which varies in intensity.

colleagues
Other people working in your establishment who may include professional, support and volunteer staff. It may include people within the same profession.

colostrum
The thick creamy milk produced by the breasts and available immediately after birth, rich in *proteins* and *antibodies*. There is no artificial replacement.

colour vision defects
The inability to recognise some colours, often an inability to distinguish between red and green.

comfort object
See *transitional object*.

communication
The ability to express oneself in gesture, speech and writing, and the ability to understand others.

community healthcare
Care carried out in the community by the *Primary Health Care team* as opposed to care in hospital.

community nurseries
Often started on large estates where the provision of a *nursery* is a focal point for young parents who may be feeling isolated, or for certain ethnic groups who wish their children to be exposed to their *cultural values*.

complications
A disease or condition occurring as a consequence of another disease such as *orchitis* (a complication of *mumps*).

compulsory care order
A child is placed in the care of the local authority, and the responsibility for the child, who is not necessarily removed from home, is shared between the local authority and the parents. The order can last until the child is 18.

concept
A general idea, a developed *schema*, and the result of learning and absorbing information.

concrete operations
According to *Piaget*, the third stage of *cognitive*

development, during which children develop the ability to think logically about things happening in the present.

conditioning
A process by which a response is reinforced, by the repetition of a certain stimulus.

conductive education
A holistic teaching and learning system designed to enable children and adults with *disabilities* to function more independently.

conductive hearing *impairment*
Sound waves are unable to pass through the eardrum or the eardrum is prevented from vibrating through the middle ear. It may be caused by a blockage of the outer ear, swollen adenoids or *otitis media*.

confidentiality
Entrusted with private information concerning a child or a family that is not divulged to anyone unless it is in the best interests of the child. Each employment setting will have rules to control the spread of private information so as to confine such information only to those who need to know, protecting and meeting the needs of the child.

conformity
Fitting in socially with the demands of the society or the peer group. Can be dangerous if people are discouraged from questioning regimes; for example the Germans conforming to the Nazi ethos in the 1930s and 1940s.

congenital
Any condition existing from birth or perhaps resulting from the birth process itself.

congenital dislocation of hip
A looseness of the hip joint so that the hip is either dislocated all the time or slips in and out of its socket. It can be detected by routine examination during the *neonatal* period.

congenital malformation
Any condition or *syndrome* that may exist at or from the time of birth. Congenital malformations range from minor skin conditions to major conditions such as *spina bifida*.

conjunctivitis
Infection or inflammation of the eye.

consent forms
In most educational and daycare establishments, parents/carers are asked to give signed consent if the staff intend taking the children off the premises, for example for swimming or for an outing. Parents/carers will also have to give written consent to *immunisation* and surgical procedures.

conservation
A *Piagetian* term to describe the awareness that two objects that are equal in volume, length, weight or amount remain equal in spite of the appearance being changed. For example, two similar balls of clay remain the same amount, even if one is re-shaped into a sausage shape.

consistency of care
The care of young children should be consistent: undertaken by the same people or person on as continuous a basis as possible.

constipation
Infrequent bowel movements and uncomfortable hard *stools* causing pain. It is important to remember that the 'emptying' *reflex* has a different pattern in different people.

construction
Describes the small and large equipment used in the *pre-school* for making models and buildings, for example bricks and blocks, Lego and so on.

consultative
See *management styles*.

consumer
The child being cared for and educated.

contagious
The spread of disease by direct or indirect personal contact, rather than in air or water.

contract of employment
In every employment, there should be a written contract stating salary, holiday entitlement, income tax, insurance and National Insurance liability, together with pension and maternity rights, and statutory sick pay. It should also show the hours and days of employment.

contusion
Injury caused, sometimes without breaking the skin, by the crushing of body tissue resulting in bruises.

convalescence
The period of recovery following an illness, injury or surgery.

convergent thinking

Thinking aimed at finding the one 'right' answer to a problem. Most children are now encouraged to think in a more creative and divergent way, sometimes called *lateral thinking*, first described by Edward de Bono.

convulsion

A fit or seizure caused by unusual nervous activity in the brain. A sudden attack of repeated involuntary muscular contractions and relaxations. Contractions may be *tonic*, continued contractions, or *clonic* (see *tonic/clonic seizure*), alternating contractions and relaxations resulting in jerking movements. See *epilepsy* and *febrile convulsion*.

co-operative play

A group of children planning some project together in a mutually supportive manner.

core subjects

Those educational subjects that have to be taught in schools, according to the *National Curriculum*.

cot death

See *sudden infant death syndrome*

coryza

A head cold or the common cold.

cough

A *reflex* response to remove irritation from the lungs. It is the mechanism for clearing the airways of excess *mucus*.

cradle cap

A crusty brown scalp seen in babies, which can be dry or greasy, often around the area of the anterior *fontanelle*. Associated with *seborrhoeic eczema*.

cradle play

Describes the baby playing in the crib, perhaps with his or her feet, or looking at a mobile.

creative play

Includes art activities and can be *structured*, but can equally well be *spontaneous* and/or *imaginative*.

creativity

Bringing into existence something original. It has been said that human beings are universally creative, but that if creativity is not valued in young children, it can be stifled and die. Creativity includes the ability to invent and research and select a wide range of materials, tools, and instruments. Creativity also includes imagination, feelings and ideas that lead to an understanding of art, music, drama, dance, stories and *imaginative play*.

crèche

A group of children of any age, looked after in a safe place for a short time to allow the parent/carer some time without a child so as to, for example, shop, or attend a hospital appointment or a conference.

critical period

A particular time in a child's development when an event has its greatest impact. (Sometimes called sensitive period.)

Crohn's disease

Chronic relapsing inflammatory disease of the bowel.

croup

One form of obstructed breathing caused by a narrowing of the larynx due to *infection*. Breathing is noisy and difficult with a characteristic sound known as stridor or croup.

crying

Communication to express a need for attention, or a strong emotion such as fear, anger, frustration or pain. The main form of communication in young babies.

culture

The customs, values, civilisation, and achievements of a particular group of people.

curd

A substance formed from the clotting of milk and used in making cheese or eaten as a food.

curriculum

A course of study. The way that children learn as well as what they learn, encompassing their whole experience and influencing all *areas of development*.

curriculum vitae (cv)

A written summary of one's career used in seeking employment.

customer

See *client/customer*.

cyanosis

Blueness of the skin.

cyst

An abnormal fluid-filled swelling.

cystic fibrosis

A *genetic* condition where secretions in the lungs and digestive system are thicker, stickier and more salty than is usual, resulting in damage to these systems. It is found in children of north European descent. It is a life threatening condition, but the symptoms can be managed by *physiotherapy* and medication. *Genetic counselling* is available.

D

dairy foods

Milk, butter, cream, cheese, and yoghurt. May come from cows, goats or sheep.

data

A collection of observations, measurements, statistics and facts; **or** the information acted upon by a computer program.

data protection

Legal safeguards for individuals, relating to information concerning them stored on computer.

day nursery

See *nursery class* and *nursery school*.

daycare

Provided for newborn to five-year-olds, often between the hours of 7.30am and 6pm, or for less time if it suits the parent/carer. The care can be run by *social services*, *workplace*s, private and *voluntary organisations*. The fees are often subsidised.

deciduous teeth

The first set of 'milk' teeth, 20 teeth that have erupted by three years. Will start to fall out by six years.

deficiency disorders

Resulting from a diet lacking certain nutrients, generally specific *vitamins* and *minerals*. For example, *anaemia* from lack of *iron*, *rickets* from lack of vitamin D and neural tube defects from lack of folic acid are all deficiency disorders.

dehydration

To lose water from the body, indicated by sunken eyes, wrinkled skin, and dry mouth and, in babies, a sunken anterior *fontanelle*.

democratic

See *management styles*.

dentition

The arrangement, type and number of teeth, the process of teething.

deregistration

See *child protection review*.

dermis

Inner layer of skin.

desirable outcomes

Set by the government, and linked with the funding of education for four-year-olds. Children should achieve desirable outcomes in personal and *social development*, language and *literacy*, *mathematics*, *creative development*, *physical development* and knowledge and understanding of the world, before starting compulsory education.

development

The acquisition of new skills, ideas, and attitudes that lead to progressive change.

development checks

Standardised tests used to check all *areas of development* in childhood, carried out in the *health centre*, school, and doctor's surgery or at home.

development of social skills

The way a child learns to relate to other people and to act in a way appropriate to his or her *society*.

developmental norms

Recognised patterns of *development* that children are expected to follow in sequence. They indicate ranges of normality.

developmental stages

See Appendix A: Developmental norms

deviant behaviour

Behaviour that varies from the standard of *behaviour* expected in the *society*. Usually describes behaviour that verges on the criminal, such as vandalism or theft.

dexterity

Smooth, rapid or skilful movement, usually of arms, hands and fingers.

diabetes insipidus

A deficiency of the pituitary gland, resulting in a disorder of water *metabolism* characterised by excessive thirst and output of unconcentrated urine.

diabetes mellitus

An inability to produce insulin that controls the amount of sugar or glucose released into the blood stream. It is potentially life threatening. The aim is to manage the blood glucose level. With hyperglycaemia it is too high, with hypoglycaemia it is too low.

dialects

The particular language of an area; for example, the Scots speak certain words in a different way from the English.

diarrhoea

Frequency of loose or watery *stools*. It is usually due to *infection*.

didactic

Meant to instruct. Didactic materials are those which have to be used in a certain very exact way, not allowing for the imagination. See *Montessori*.

dieticians

Professionals, trained in *nutrition*, who advise people with eating disorders on how to eat in a healthier fashion. They are also the experts on *special diets* for sick people and for those with *allergic* reactions to some foods.

digit

A finger or toe.

diphtheria

An extremely dangerous disease that has been wiped out in the UK by *immunisation*. The characteristic symptom is the membrane that grows on the tonsils. Swelling of the throat may become so severe that breathing is prevented.

disability

Any restriction, or lack (resulting from *impairment*) of ability to perform an activity in the manner or within the range considered normal for a human being (WHO, 1980).

disability, complex conditions

The causes of these conditions are various and complicated. They influence several developmental areas, and need *consistency of care* and management. They include *Down's syndrome, fragile X syndrome, sensory impairment, spina bifida, cerebral palsy* and *learning difficulty*.

disability, conditions affecting communication and control

It is sometimes difficult to establish a cause, but these conditions result in children finding difficulty in controlling and directing speech, *behaviour*, relationships and movement and include *dyslexia, dysphaxia, autism*, speech and *communication impairment, emotional* and *behavioural* difficulties.

disability, legislation

The recent main acts concerning disability are: Warnock 1978; *Children Act, 1989;* Code of Practice, 1994; Education Acts, 1981, 1988 and 1993; NHS and Community Care Act, 1990; and Disability Discrimination Acts 1995 and 1997.

disability, physical conditions

These are conditions where you will need some knowledge of *anatomy* and *physiology* to understand the causes. They require regular medical supervision and often the use of medicines to control and minimise the effects. They include *epilepsy, asthma* and *eczema, diabetes, HIV* and *AIDS, coeliac disease, haemophilia, cystic fibrosis, sickle cell, thalassaemia*, and *muscular dystrophy*.

disability, therapies

Children with disabilities will need and respond to many treatments, including *Portage, soundbeam, respite care, patterning, conductive education, physiotherapy, speech therapy, occupational therapy*.

disciplinary procedure

A method of investigating and dealing with a complaint against a person in employment or on a course of study.

discipline

Management of *behaviour*, initially exercised by others (parents and teachers), but eventually leading to self-control.

disclosure

The term used to describe when a child confides in someone that he or she has been *abused*.

discrimination

Treating certain people or groups of people in an unfair manner based solely on *prejudice*.

disinfection

To destroy *pathogenic micro-organisms* or their *toxins*, generally by the use of chemicals, or in some cases by boiling. Disinfectant is harmful to body tissue.

disinfest

To dispose of vermin.

display

Putting children's work on show raises the sense of self-worth and confidence in the children, as the work is seen to be valued. Work should be displayed in an *aesthetic* manner.

divergent thinking

A *creative* way of problem solving, sometimes described as *lateral thinking*.

domestic play

Pretending to make cups of tea and doing domestic chores, often taking place in the home corner or at home.

domestic violence

Aggressive behaviour that occurs in households across the *class* range. The *perpetrator* of violence is not necessarily a drunk, or a victim of abuse but uses a system of control to manipulate the weaker partner. The abuser is often charming when not being violent.

dominant genes

One or other of the parents will be affected by the *gene*, and each of their children has a 50 per cent chance of inheriting the condition, which may be a disorder, such as *achondroplasia* or a family feature, such as colour of eyes.

Down's syndrome

A genetic condition resulting from the presence of an extra chromosome. Children with *Down's syndrome* will share some physical characteristics, will have a *learning difficulty* and may have a range of associated physical problems: heart, respiratory and sensory.

drop in centres

Opened mainly in inner city areas, they are centres where parents/carers can 'drop in' with their babies and toddlers, and make friends while the children *play*.

DTP triple *vaccine*

Given by injection, this protects against *diphtheria*, *tetanus*, and *whooping cough* (*pertussis*).

Duchenne muscular dystrophy

An inherited condition resulting in a fault in a *protein* in muscle fibre – dystrophin. There is increasing muscular weakness and breakdown of muscle cells.

dysentery

The term describing a number of intestinal diseases resulting in fever, abdominal cramps, and severe *diarrhoea*.

dyslexia

A condition affecting areas of reading, spelling and written language, resulting in a specific *learning difficulty*. *Intelligence quotient* (IQ) is generally normal.

dysphasia

Impaired co-ordination of speech.

dyspraxia

Difficulty or immaturity in the organisation of movement affecting *gross* and *fine motor development*. Normal range of *cognition*.

E

early experience

Some people believe that early experiences are the most important in influencing a child's all round development. The Jesuits (a religious group) famously said, 'Give me a child until he is seven, and he is mine for life'.

early neonatal mortality

Deaths in the first six days of life.

early years development plan (EYDP)

All local authorities are expected to submit a plan to the DfEE demonstrating how a good quality nursery place can be provided for each eligible four-year-old whose parents want one.

early years forums

A mechanism for the local authority to establish links, and consult with parents and the private and voluntary sector. People and organisations that provide services for children under eight years should be included, as well as the wider community. One of their tasks may be to draw up an *early years development plan*.

ectopic pregnancy

A pregnancy occurring outside the *uterus* usually within a Fallopian tube.

eczema

Patches on the skin that are dry and extremely irritating. The skin may become inflamed and cracked and more vulnerable to *infection*.

education services

The private and public provision of education. The *statutory* requirement is for five to sixteen year-olds, but there are many services for pre-schoolers and adults.

educational neglect
Refers to children who lack stimulation in their *environment* and may find difficulty in achieving at school or nursery.

educational programmes
Some pre-schools follow special programmes. *High Scope* is a programme where the children are expected to choose their own activity for the session and then report back on what took place; *Montessori* is named after the famous doctor and educationalist, where the programme is structured, using specialised *didactic* equipment; and *Steiner*, where the programme is to educate the whole child, has an emphasis on spirituality.

educational psychologist
A professional trained to assess children's intellectual ability and potential, who may recommend placing children in *special schools*.

ego
A term used in *Freudian* psychology, describing a sense of one's own individuality and worth.

egocentricity
Piaget describes this as an inability to see another's point of view. He stated that children younger than seven could only see their own point of view (the three mountains research), but more recently children as young as four have de-centred using more relevant equipment.

embryo
The baby during the first three months of pregnancy.

emergency protection order
Intended for use in real emergencies when children might suffer harm. Anyone can apply to the court for such an order, which lasts for a maximum of eight days.

emergent writing
Children who have grasped the concept that the marks on paper represent words, often make marks themselves, and tell you what they represent.

emotional abuse
Exposed to constant criticism, hostility, and lack of affection and warmth. There may be rejection or extreme over-protection. It results in poor *self-esteem* and lack of confidence. It can occur with any age group.

emotional development
The stages a child passes through, from utter dependence to full autonomy.

emotional neglect
The parents/carers may withdraw love from a child and fail to provide an *environment* filled with warmth, interest and love.

empathy
The way in which one identifies with and fully understands another person's emotions.

employment of children
The law lays down firm guidelines as to the ages at which people can do certain jobs. Children are often *exploited* by being asked to do jobs for which they are too young, working too many hours, and being paid far below the going adult rate.

employment opportunities
There are many opportunities for qualified childcare practitioners, in the private home setting as nannies and child-minders, in educational establishments, in *daycare* settings, in hospitals' *obstetric* wards, *health centres* and Special Care Baby Units (SCBUs), in *playgroups*, and in many different types of *crèche*. The growth of leisure provision has resulted in new opportunities, such as in shopping and sports centres.

employment protection
Legislation to protect members of staff in the workplace, which includes equal pay, access to medical reports, *race relations*, *disability*, harassment, health and safety, and *sex discrimination*.

empowerment
Giving children a feeling of power. *Imaginative play* involving superheroes and super-heroines or *role play* as policemen and policewomen helps to empower children.

empty calories
Sugar, sweet drinks, sweets that provide *calories* (energy) for the body, but contain no other nutrients.

enabling
To act or respond in a way that allows someone else to achieve.

encephalitis
Inflammation of the brain, usually as a result of a viral *infection*.

encopresis
Frequent faecal soiling that is age inappropriate.

endemic
Describes a disease that is always present in a

particular area of the world, such as malaria in some parts of Africa.

eneurisis
Bedwetting. Used to describe a condition in children who show no sign of becoming dry at night by the age of four, or who start to wet the bed again after becoming dry.

environment
The physical surroundings, conditions, relationships and circumstances in which a person lives.

enzymes
Proteins produced by living cells that act as catalysts accelerating and promoting a chemical change. In the digestive system their function is to speed up the rate at which food is digested. Examples include pepsin in the stomach which digests protein, and amylase, found in pancreatic juice and saliva, which digests starch.

epidemic
Occurs when a disease spreads rapidly and infects large numbers of people, then disappears until the next outbreak.

epidermis
Outer layer of skin.

epidural anaesthesia
An injection of local anaesthetic into the space around the spinal cord.

epiglottis
Flap of tissue at the back of the throat.

epilepsy
Caused by an interruption in the chemical activity in the nerve cells of the brain responsible for consciousness, awareness, movement and posture, resulting in a fit or seizure. See *tonic/clonic seizure (grand mal)* and *absences (petit mal)*.

episiotomy
A small cut in the *perineum* to enlarge the vagina, to facilitate the birth process.

epistaxis
Nose bleed.

equal opportunities
Along with other professionals, childcare practitioners need to recognise that no member of *society* should be *discriminated* against because of his or her *gender*, *race*, *disability*, *culture*, religion, age, *class* or *sexual orientation*. Opportunities must be offered to all on an equal basis.

Erikson, Eric H. (1902–1994)
Born in Germany of Danish parents. Leading psychoanalyst and researcher into human development. Extended *Freud*'s psychoanalytical theory to include the influence of *culture* and *society* on personality. His theory of stages was based on 'the eight stages of man'.

ethics
A code of moral values, governed by rules and principles, that may be held by a group of people in a profession or by an individual.

ethnic
Refers to a particular racial group.

ethnocentricity
The belief that the ethnic group to which you belong is superior to any other.

ethologist
A person who studies the science of animal behaviour, viewed in the wild, extended to include human beings by observing them in their natural habitat, such as the *pre-school*, or in the *family*.

evaluation
The term used by childcare practitioners to assess and *appraise observations* and *activities*, so as to plan for the future.

event sample
An *observation* that tries to discover why a child is behaving in an *aggressive* manner. Over a week or so, a number of *observations* are carried out. Each time the child acts aggressively the *data* is examined to see if there is an emerging pattern to the *behaviour*, for example, was the child provoked, or is the same child the victim each time, or do the attacks happen at the same time of day?

excretion
Removal of waste from the body by urination and defecation.

experiential learning
Learning through one's own experience, not just from books.

exploitation of children
Children may be unfairly treated by being exposed to illegal *employment*, *child prostitution*, *sex tourism*, *paedophiles*, *family abductions*.

exploration of the outside world

As young children venture outside their family home, they learn about different *environments* and different value systems. Most children adapt very quickly to outside stimulation (such as going to *pre-school*), and learn a great deal.

extended day provision

Pre-school children are cared for before school starts and after school ends, mainly to help working mothers. The provisions are often run by *social services* and a small fee is charged to provide tea and/or breakfast. The children are usually looked after in a different part of the building, in a homely atmosphere.

extended family

The family outside the *nuclear family* of parents and children, to include grandparents, aunts, uncles, nephews, nieces and so on.

eye contact

Gazing at another, often without words, but maintaining contact with the eyes only. Shown in *bonding*. Withholding eye contact is seen as a negative factor in *non-verbal communication*.

Eysenck, Hans (1916–1997)

German-born British psychologist. Best known for his controversial work on personality and intelligence, claiming that *genetic* factors play a large part in the differences between people.

F

failure to thrive

This occurs when children fail to gain weight or to grow and achieve their expected weight and height. A child, who has no medical or physical reason not to develop normally, may fail to thrive resulting from a negative relationship with the parent/carer. This is more likely to be picked up in the younger age group, when children are regularly monitored and attending *health centres*.

family

The group of people, generally related, but may include friends, who are significant and important to a child. See *extended family*, *nuclear family*.

family abduction

When a family unit breaks up, there may be disputes between the parents as to the custody of the children. If these are not resolved one parent might forcibly remove the children, away from the family home. This can be most traumatic, and is a form of *child abuse*.

family grouping

See *vertical grouping*.

fats (lipids)

Provide warmth and energy for the body, store some *vitamins*, protect body organs and enhance the flavour of food. Fats are divided into saturated fats, which are solid and mainly animal; unsaturated fats, which are liquid from vegetables and fish oil; and polyunsaturated fats, mainly from plant sources and low in *cholesterol*.

febrile

A raised temperature.

febrile convulsion

A fit caused by a sudden high temperature in a child, that results in unconsciousness, twitching and shaking, the eyes may roll, and froth may come out of the mouth. It is followed by a period of sleep.

feral

Refers to animals in the wild, often cats that have been left to die. This has on occasion happened to children, who have been succoured by animals. These children may survive but their development is always severely retarded.

fetal alcohol syndrome

A condition in *newborn* babies, caused by an excessive intake of alcohol by the mother during pregnancy, that results in various defects and is characterised by certain facial features.

fetus

The baby from three months of pregnancy to birth.

fibre

Found in plant foods, it contains no nourishment for humans as it cannot be digested. It adds bulk to the diet and aids digestion. It is also known as roughage.

fine motor development

The development of manipulative skills, involving hand–eye co-ordination.

fistula

An abnormal connection between two hollow body organs or between a hollow organ and the skin.

fit
See *convulsion*.

fit person
When registering a person to care for children under eight years the local authority has a duty to ensure that he or she is suitable. All people living or working on the premises have to be 'fit'. The local authority will look at experience, qualifications and training, ability to provide warmth and *consistency of care*, awareness of *multicultural* issues and *equal opportunities*, physical and mental health and a background free from criminal conviction.

fleas
See *parasites*.

flow and movement charts
Charts showing how children might move around the classroom or the playground: a form of *observation*.

fluoride
A *mineral* found in some water, bones of fish or added to water, toothpaste, or drops. It makes tooth enamel more resistant to decay. See *caries*.

fomites
Inanimate objects, such as toys, dishes and clothing that may harbour *pathogens* and transmit *infection*.

fontanelles (soft spots)
Gaps between the flat bones of the skull that allow moulding during labour. The anterior fontanelle is at the front (top) of the head, the posterior near the crown (back) of the head.

food allergy
The body's rejection of a food, sometimes causing an *allergic* reaction.

food groups
Foods grouped together according to the main nutrient they provide. *Proteins, carbohydrates, vitamins, minerals* and *fibre, fats* and oils.

food intolerance
The body's inability to digest or absorb a specific food.

food poisoning
The body's response to contaminated food, generally short lived; symptoms may include *diarrhoea, vomiting* and abdominal pain.

forceps delivery
The use of instruments with curved ends that fit and lock around the baby's head. Gentle traction is used to deliver the baby under local anaesthetic.

fore milk
The milk produced at the beginning of a breast-feed, high in lactose.

formal operations
According to *Piaget*, the final stage in *cognitive* ability, being able to think abstractly.

formula milk
Essential for babies who are not breast-fed. Mainly cow's milk that has been adapted by changes to the *fat* and *protein* content and with added *vitamins* and *minerals*. It may be *curd* dominant containing the protein casein, for hungrier babies, or *whey* dominant containing the protein lactalbumin which is nearer in composition to breast milk.

fortified foods
Some foods such as bread, cereals and margarine, have *vitamins* and *minerals* added to them.

foster care
Children in need of care outside their own homes, for various reasons, may be placed with a family who have been approved by the local authority as suitable to bring up the child in the short or long term.

fragile X syndrome
An inherited condition passed on by the X chromosome, resulting in *learning difficulties* and some physical characteristics.

frenulum
The folds of mucus membrane that attach the upper and lower lips to the gums.

Freud, Sigmund (1856–1939)
Austrian neurologist and founder of psychoanalysis. Initially, he used hypnosis in treatment, then developed the technique of 'free association'. He believed in recovered memory, which is much criticised today.

Froebel, Frederick (1782–1852)
German educationalist. Founded the kindergarten system. Believed that *structured play* was vital to children's development.

fructarian diet
A diet based on fruit and uncooked cereals and seeds.

fungi
A *micro-organism* causing *ringworm*, athlete's foot and *thrush*.

G

games with rules
Very young children have difficulty in following games which cannot be played without rules, such as Ludo, until they reach a certain stage of *moral development*, at about four and a half years.

gastro-enteritis
This may be associated with an *infection* in the bowels or elsewhere in the body, or with *food poisoning*. The symptoms are *diarrhoea*, *vomiting*, abdominal pain and sometimes fever. There is a danger of *dehydration*.

gender
Male or female.

gene
A unit of heredity, forming part of a *chromosome*, that determines a particular characteristic in an individual.

genetic counselling
Advice and information given by skilled practitioners to parents about the possibility and probability of passing on an inherited condition.

genetics
The study of heredity and variation in *organisms*; **or** the features and constitution of a single organism, species or group.

genital stage
Freud's final stage of mature psycho-sexual development.

Gesell, Alfred L. (1880–1961)
American pioneer in *child development*, particularly early infant development.

gestation
The number of weeks a woman is pregnant prior to delivery of the baby.

gifted
Refers to exceptionally talented or intelligent children.

glue ear
A condition in which the middle ear becomes filled with fluid instead of air. It may result in partial hearing loss.

glycosuria
Sugar in the urine.

gonads
Sex organs.

grand mal
A serious form of *epilepsy* with loss of consciousness. See *tonic/clonic seizure*.

grasp reflex
The baby's fist will clench any object placed in the palm of the hand, and will support the baby's weight if fingers are placed into the palms.

graze
See *abrasion*.

grazing
The habit of constantly eating food throughout the day, to eat snacks rather than formal meals.

grievance procedure
An employment procedure to deal with a real or fancied cause for complaint by a member of staff.

gross motor development
The development of the large muscles and limbs, charting the progress of the *newborn* baby with no control, to the active child who can run, hop, skip, climb and jump. *Vigorous physical play* helps to promote the development of *gross motor* skills.

group dynamics
A term used by social psychologists to describe how certain groups of people come together, make relationships and decisions, interact and develop.

group play
Playing in a group.

growth
An increase in size that is measurable. Linear growth is the length of the baby's body or the height of a child. There should be a consistent weight gain. Regular measurements of the *head circumference* indicates the growth of the brain within the skull. These measurements are taken at birth, and used as the baseline for future measurements. The figures should be plotted on a *percentile chart*.

growth spurt
A sudden increase in height, weight and *head circumference*. It may be seen to occur after a period of illness or later, during adolescence.

Guthrie test
A blood test to screen for *phenylketonuria* usually carried out within days of the birth for all babies in the UK.

H

haematuria
Blood in the urine.

haemophilia
A blood disorder, inherited from the mother, that affects only boys. There is a defect in the clotting mechanism of the blood, resulting in excessive bruising and prolonged bleeding causing pain and swellings. In the most severely affected there is spontaneous bleeding into joints and muscles.

halal
Meat from animals killed according to Islamic tradition.

halitosis
Offensive breath. Rare in children but may be caused by poor oral and dental *hygiene* or severe *tonsillitis*.

hand, foot and mouth syndrome
A viral *infection* resulting in a *rash* of greyish white blistering spots with a red halo, seen on the tongue, palms of the hands, and on the sides of the feet. **Not** to be confused with the animal disease, foot and mouth.

hare lip
The split in the lip, which can occur in association with *cleft palate*.

hazards
Dangers, such as long flexes on kettles, and splinters in wooden blocks, that may contribute to accidents.

head circumference
Measurement of the maximum circumference of the skull. It is measured at birth and at regular health checks to confirm *growth* of the brain.

head lag
Describes the way the head falls back when the baby is pulled into a sitting position.

health
A state of complete mental, physical, and social well-being, and not merely the absence of disease or infirmity (WHO).

health centres
Premises providing health care for a local community and usually having a group practice, nurses, *health visitors*, community midwives, *child health centres* and perhaps other services such as *speech therapy*, dental care and chiropody.

health promotion
The process of enabling people to control and improve their health. To achieve this, individuals or groups must be able to realise their aspirations, to satisfy needs, and to change or cope with their *environment*. It is not the responsibility of the *health services* alone, and goes beyond healthy lifestyles to look at other ways of promoting well-being (adapted from the Ottawa Charter 1986).

health screening
A test or examination for a particular disease or condition that allows it to be cured or treated. If detected early permanent damage or *disability* may be prevented. Health professionals need to be trained to carry out and interpret the tests correctly. The tests are offered to large groups of the population.

health services
The provision of community and hospital care, to prevent disease, diagnose illness and provide treatment.

health surveillance
To watch and observe children closely, regular *assessments* of *growth*, *health*, and developmental progress are made at certain ages by professional workers.

health visitors
Professionals, who are also nurses, who visit babies, young children and the elderly in their own homes. Members of the *Primary Health Care team*.

heritage language
The language learnt in the home.

hernia
A bulge of tissue protruding through an abnormal opening between muscles.

herpes simplex
A cold sore around the nose or nostril caused by a *virus*. They lie dormant, and tend to flare up with each new cold.

heterosexism

Can be an individual or an institutional response to *homosexual* behaviour, regarding it as an inferior state. It reinforces the myth of heterosexuality as the superior *sexual orientation.*

heterosexuality

Emotional and sexual relationship between people of the opposite *gender.*

Hib vaccine

An injection that protects against *infection* by the *bacteria* Haemophilus influenzae type b, which can cause *septicaemia, pneumonia,* or *meningitis.*

High Scope

See *educational programmes.*

hindmilk

Follows the *foremilk* with the *let-down reflex.* It is high in *fat* and *calories* to satisfy the baby's hunger and ensure *growth.*

histogram

A statistical analysis, similar to a *bar chart,* sometimes used to describe *data* graphically in *observations.*

holistic approach

An approach to the care of a child, where the total needs are recognised and met. A holistic education is one that educates the whole child, in all the areas of *child development,* not just in basic *cognitive* skills. The *curriculum* would include the arts, music, and physical activity among others.

home visit

A visit made by a member of the *pre-school, daycare* or *infant school* team to the home of a child on the waiting list. It is helpful for the family to meet the member of staff, and have someone to relate to immediately the child starts, and for the establishment to be on less formal terms with the parents/carers than would be the case if the visit had not taken place. It is also an opportunity to discuss in *partnership* any *challenging behaviour* a child might present, any *special diets* and any favourite words used by the child that adults might not otherwise understand.

homophobia

Fear of *homosexuality* in relation to self, which produces disgust, and contempt for and hatred of lesbians and gay men.

homosexuality

The emotional and sexual relationship between people of the same *gender,* known as gay if they are men and lesbian if they are women.

horizontal grouping

A term sometimes used in schools to define age grouping and refers to all the children of the same age being in the same class, whatever their ability.

hormones

Chemical substances, produced in the endocrine glands, and taken by the bloodstream to various parts of the body where they have a specific function, such as insulin that controls the level of blood sugar, and prolactin that stimulates the secretion of breast milk.

hospice

A nursing home that specialises in caring for the *terminally ill.* There are now several hospices for children, where a *multi-disciplinary team* will support children and their *families* at home as well as in the hospice.

human immunodeficiency virus (HIV)

A *virus* that attacks the body's immune system, particularly white blood cells (CD4 or T-helpercells). There may be no sign of ill health for many years.

hydrocephalus

An abnormal build-up of fluid surrounding the brain, resulting in an enlarged head in children, whose skull bones have not yet grown together. It is usually *congenital,* but may result from *trauma* leading to compression of the brain. It is often associated with *spina bifida.*

hygiene

Concerned with the maintenance of *health,* promoting clean and healthy practices and *routines.* The childcare practitioner is important as a role model in setting standards in personal hygiene, and *health promotion.*

hypermetropia

Distant objects are seen clearly, those nearby are blurred. Opposite to *myopia.*

hypospadias

A condition in which the urethra opens onto the under surface of the penis.

hypothermia

An abnormally low body temperature, generally through exposure to cold weather. Babies are very vulnerable, as they are unable to generate heat for themselves. They can also look deceptively healthy with this condition.

hypothesis
A proposition made as a basis for reasoning, without the assumption of truth.

hypothyroidism
See *thyroid deficiency*.

I

imaginative play
Children imagine fantastic situations, like living on the moon, and what might happen if the dinosaurs were still on the earth. It is helpful in developing *creativity* and imagination.

imitative play
An early type of *play* particularly enjoyed by toddlers, when they copy others, usually their parent/carer.

immature language
Some children speak in an immature way, having difficulty in pronouncing certain sounds. This will right itself in time, and the general advice is to ignore immature speech, being sure always to respond to the child clearly, and with proper grammatical forms.

immune system
A natural body response for recognising and destroying invading *micro-organisms* or foreign tissue. Based on the white blood cells.

immunisation
See *vaccination*.

immunisation programme
Being given protection against certain diseases by participating in a schedule offered at a national level by GPs, and *health centres*. The programme aims to protect the whole community as well as individual children. See *vaccination*.

immunity
Resistance developed by the body against a disease. It may be achieved naturally by contracting a disease and developing *antibodies* or artificially by *vaccination*.

impairment
See *disability*.

impetigo
A *contagious* skin *infection* that may affect healthy skin or be a *complication* of another skin condition. It is often seen in the nose and mouth area with pustules that rupture and form thick yellow crusts. Medical advice should be sought.

in situ
In the natural or original position.

incest
Sexual intercourse between two people who are too closely related to marry. It includes parents and children.

inclusiveness
An *environment* or establishment that can be used by all children, including those with *disabilities*, can be described as inclusive.

incubation period
The period of time between the original *infection* and when the *symptoms* appear.

indicators of abuse
Abuse may be suspected by the *behaviour* of the child, the physical appearance of the child, or by *disclosure*.

induction of labour
Starting labour artificially either by rupturing the membranes or giving *hormones*.

infancy
The first year of life.

infant mortality
Deaths under one year of age.

infant school
An educational establishment for children aged five to seven years.

infection
Invasion of the body by *pathogenic micro-organisms*.

infectious hepatitis
Due to a *virus* that spreads through the body but mainly damages the liver. Of the two forms, A and B, B is more severe but rare in childhood. A third form, C, has recently been described.

infestation
Invasion of *parasites* living on or in a human host.

ingestion

To take food or liquid into the body.

inhalation of micro-organisms

A very common cause of infection is taking *micro-organisms* in through the nose and throat. This is sometimes knows as droplet *infection*.

inhalers (puffers)

Equipment used by children over five years of age with asthma, to prevent or relieve attacks of asthma. The aerosol canister fits into the inhaler that is then inserted into the mouth. The child has to co-ordinate pressing the canister and inhaling, allowing the medicine to be taken directly into the lungs.

inhaling

To take breath in through the nose and mouth to the lungs.

inoculations

When *organisms* enter the body by cuts or *abrasions* to the skin. It can include the process of introducing a *vaccine* to the body by injection.

insurance

A payment of a sum of money to protect against certain situations occurring. All daycare establishments must be covered by employers' liability insurance against claims by employees for injury or disease. Anyone who provides daycare either in an institution or privately should consider holding public liability insurance. This covers legal liability for omissions or acts that cause injury or disease to third parties. It is also possible to insure against, for example, having twins, or bad weather at the annual school fete.

intelligence quotient (IQ)

A score calculated by dividing a person's mental age by his or her chronological age, and multiplying by 100. When used sensitively it can be useful in describing a person's potential ability.

interaction

See *adult interaction*.

interpersonal relationships

Reciprocal relationships between people.

intervention

See *adult intervention*.

intussusception

Occurs when a segment of bowel is pulled down the centre of the bowel causing a blockage of the intestine.

iron

A *mineral* essential in the diet to form haemoglobin that carries oxygen to all body tissues.

irradiation of food

The exposure of food to gamma rays to reduce the number of *pathogenic organisms*, control *infestation*, and delay ripening and sprouting. All food treated in this way should be labelled.

Isaacs, Susan (1885–1948)

Follower of *Freud*, believing in the influence of *early experiences*. Set up a school where children were expected to learn by discovery. Did not believe in *autocratic* rules, but allowed for emotional expression.

isolated behaviour

Worrying behaviour in some children who find it impossible to develop relationships and so do not interact with their *peer group*, refusing to join in with even one other child in any activity.

isolation

To separate a person from others to prevent the spread of *infection*; **or** describes the behaviour of some children (see *isolated behaviour*).

J

jaundice

A yellow discoloration of the skin, caused by an excess in the bloodstream of the chemical bilirubin, a natural waste product of the continuous breakdown of red cells in the blood.

jealousy

Feeling resentful of others in rivalry for love, possessions and attention. *Sibling rivalry* describes brothers and sisters vying for the affection of a parent or carer.

job description

A formal written statement of the duties and responsibilities required by a particular job.

job search

The process of seeking employment, by responding to advertisements or approaching agencies.

joule

A measurement of food energy.

Jung, Carl G. (1875–1961)

Swiss psychiatrist. Worked with *Freud* for many years, but became increasingly critical on the emphasis that Freud put on psychosexual reasons for neurosis. Developed his own school, introducing the words 'extrovert' and 'introvert' to describe outgoing and reserved personality types.

K

Kanner's syndrome

See *autism*.

key worker

Generally in daycare establishments. The key worker is the person who has responsibility for the overall care of a child, writing *observations*, providing *activities*, keeping *records* and liaising with parents.

Kitemark

The official mark of quality and reliability on equipment approved by the British Standards Institute.

Koplik spots

White spots seen in the inside of cheeks in the early stages of *measles*.

kosher

Preparation of food and slaughtering of animals according to Judaic law. Several animal foods are prohibited, and milk foods are not prepared or eaten with meat.

L

labelling

To categorise a person by using labels such as 'handicapped' or 'sub-normal' is not useful as the label focuses on the *disability* only, and tells nothing of how he or she is coping with that disability.

lactation

The production of breast milk.

laissez faire

See *management styles*.

language acquisition device (LAD)

The inborn ability to learn a language, as described by *Noam Chomsky* (1972).

language delay

Some children learn to speak and to understand language later than others do. There is usually no need to worry, but language delay can point to *learning difficulties*.

language development

Describes the way that language develops through encouragement, and by others *listening*, promoting and extending experiences. See Appendix B.

lanugo

Fine hair that covers the face and body of the *fetus*.

lap play

The baby playing with an adult, lying in his or her lap.

late neonatal mortality

Deaths in the first seven to twenty-seven days of life.

latency period

Freud calls the period of comparative calm between six years and puberty, the latency period.

lateral thinking

See *convergent thinking*.

learning

Changes in *behaviour* that result from experience, and acquiring new knowledge and skills.

learning by discovery

Learning by doing, a theory first put into practice by *Susan Isaacs*, whose school encouraged children to find out by experimenting rather than *didactic* methods.

learning difficulty

Can be mild, moderate, severe or profound. There are various causes, some examples of which are *Down's syndrome, fragile X syndrome, autism, speech/language* and *sensory impairment*.

learning environment

Describes an *environment* that is stimulating and exciting, offering opportunities for learning new skills and for exploration.

let-down reflex

The interaction between the baby sucking at the nipple, the breast nerves stimulating the mother's brain and the pituitary gland to release the *hormone* prolactin to make milk, and oxytocin to contract breast muscles pushing milk down the ducts to the nipple.

lethargy
An abnormal lack of energy.

leukaemia
Cancer of the white blood cells.

lice
See *parasites*.

light for dates
Babies born below the expected weight for their period of *gestation*.

listening
In educational terms, the ability to actively listen often encourages a child to carry on a conversation. A good listener, who does not try to monopolise the give and take of conversation, will give a child confidence and a feeling of self-worth.

listeriosis
An *organism* found in pâté and soft cheeses that can damage the *fetus*.

literacy
The ability to read and write. Literacy is attained in many ways, using reading schemes (look and say, phonics, real books) and other techniques. It is hoped *emergent writing* will lead to legible writing, and reading schemes to an independent enjoyment of books.

locomotion
The ability to move. It generally describes the process from birth when the baby has no head control, through the stages of gaining control, sitting, crawling, pulling to stand, and finally walking.

longitudinal study
An *observation* of one child, carried out over several weeks.

low birth-weight baby
Weighing 2.5 kg (5.5 lb) or less.

M

Macmillan, Margaret (1860–1931) and Rachel (1859–1917)
American-born, but brought up in the UK. Educational reformers, they opened the first school clinic in 1908 and the first open air nursery school in 1914. Particularly involved with very poor children and in educating their mothers in *nutrition*, *health* and *learning*.

Macmillan nurses
Trained nurses who specialise in looking after *cancer* patients in their own homes, and in supporting their relatives/carers.

macro-nutrients
Foods that provide energy for the body and are needed in relatively large amounts. They are measured in grams.

Makaton
A structured signing system, used to complement speech development.

malignant
Evil; **or** may refer to a *tumour* that is uncontrollable or resistant to *therapy*.

malleable
Pliable, will respond to pressure.

malnutrition
Lack of essential nutrients in the body, it may be due to an inadequate diet, an unbalanced diet or an inability to digest foods properly.

management styles
There are four main styles: laissez faire, democratic, consultative, and autocratic. Many management styles are a mixture of two or more styles. Laissez faire refers to weak management, where the supposed leader of the team just allows the staff to do as they think best. Democratic describes a style with a strong leader, who keeps the staff fully informed of all proposed changes and plans. Consultative refers to the team meeting often, and discussing together the best ways to approach future plans. An autocratic style describes a team where the leader makes all the decisions without telling or consulting the staff in advance.

masturbation
Stimulating the genital organs to achieve sexual pleasure, a common practice in children of both sexes causing no harm to *health* or development. The child will soon learn that it is a taboo to masturbate in public. For a few children it becomes a compulsive comfort habit.

maternity nurse
A person employed by a *family* following the birth of a new baby who will live in for a short period of time to care for the *newborn*.

mathematical activities
Activities that involve counting and recording, length and area, *capacity and volume*, measuring, time, money, sorting (sets, shape and colour), weight, numeracy and *conservation*.

maturation
The process of *growth* and development linked with the attainment of maturity.

mature milk
The name given to breast milk from about the tenth day. It looks thin and watery by comparison with the milk mixed with *colostrum* but is still appropriate to the baby's needs.

measles
A highly infectious disease caused by a *virus* that spreads through the body but affects mainly the skin and respiratory tract. It is less common since the introduction of an *immunisation programme*.

meconium
The greenish sticky faecal matter passed by the newborn infant within a few hours of birth.

medical model of disability
Labels disabled people as ill and in need of treatment and regards the *disability* as an illness. The emphasis is on a medical cause, treatment or cure. It disregards disabled people's own feelings and leaves them dependent on others.

melanoma
A dark pigmented *tumour* of the skin that may be *malignant*.

meningitis
An infection of the meninges, the protective layers next to and surrounding the brain and spinal cord. *Viruses* or *bacteria* may cause it. It is important to obtain medical aid very quickly.

metabolism
The chemical processes that occur in the body resulting in *growth*, production of energy and elimination of waste.

microcephaly
A head that is disproportionately small for the age and body size of a child.

micronutrients
Vitamins and *minerals* that do not supply energy and are needed in relatively small amounts. They are measured in milligrams and micrograms.

micro-organisms
Living matter that is too small to be seen by the human eye, such as *bacteria, fungi, viruses* and *protozea*.

minerals
Inorganic matter, found in soil and absorbed into plants. Eaten in food or in supplements, and are essential for *health*.

miscarriage
See *abortion*.

MMR vaccine
An injection to protect against *measles, mumps*, and *rubella*.

Mongolian blue spot
A bluish discoloration of the lower back, seen in babies of Asian, African and Afro-Caribbean origin. It becomes less obvious as the child grows up. It may be mistaken for bruising.

monitoring
Observations and *assessments* are made in order to have a careful record of part of the development of a child in your care. Doctors may also monitor a child about whom they are worried, using *percentile charts*, for example.

Montessori, Maria (1870–1952)
Italian doctor and educationalist, her system was originally developed for children from socially deprived backgrounds and with *disabilities*, but now has worldwide appeal. *Didactic* materials are used in Montessori schools, which have to be used in a proscribed manner.

moral development
Morality is developed in stages; obedience, naïve egoism, trying to please, understanding rules, 'sense of fairness', and finally gaining a conscience. Sensitivity and *empathy* lead to awareness and tolerance of other people's traditions, *cultures* and religions.

Moro reflex
The baby's head is held in the doctor's hand and raised a little before being released quickly. The baby's arms will stretch out with fingers curved and will then be brought back across the chest as if in an embrace.

mortality rate
The frequency or number of deaths in proportion to a population.

mother's help
He or she will work in the household to help the parent with the children and the chores. They are paid more than *au pairs* and expected to work more hours. Being untrained, they will need a certain amount of supervision, according to their experience. To make matters more muddling, the employers often refer to them as 'the *nanny*'.

motor
A term applied to nerves that relay orders from the brain to the muscles, resulting in movement.

mucus
A sticky fluid that acts as a protective lubricant coating within the four body systems that open to the outside of the body: the respiratory, digestive, urinary, and reproductive systems.

multicultural (multi-ethnic) society
Refers to the constitution of several *ethnic* groups within a society.

multicultural environment
Describes an *environment* which reflects many *cultures*, in books, posters, dressing-up clothes, home corner equipment, jigsaws, music, cooking recipes and so on.

multi-disciplinary team
A team of professionals from different disciplines working together with a common aim.

multilingualism
The ability to speak more than two languages.

multiple births
See *twins*. The increasing use of fertilisation treatment has resulted in more pregnancies where three or more children have been born.

multiple caring
The parents share the nurture of the child with other people, such as childcare practitioners, grandparents and other members of an *extended family*.

mumps
An infectious disease caused by a *virus*. The salivary glands swell, the parotid gland, in front of the ear is particularly affected. *Immunisation* is now available.

Munchausen's syndrome by proxy
Used to describe a psychological condition where a parent fabricates a child's illness, seeking many different medical opinions and treatments, and inducing *symptoms* in the child to deceive the doctors.

muscle tone
The constant state of slight contraction in the skeletal muscles that are responsible for *posture* and movement. Regular exercise is essential to maintain good muscle tone, enabling the body to feel firm not flabby.

muscular dystrophies
A group of diseases in which the muscles degenerate and weaken.

myopia (short sight)
Near objects are seen clearly, those at a distance are blurred. The opposite to *hypermetropia*.

N

naevus
Congenital abnormality of the skin presenting as a birthmark or mole.

naming systems
The appropriate oral and written forms of address for children and their families. These will vary depending on tradition, *culture* and *ethnic* background.

nanny
A trained or untrained person, who is employed to care for children in the home setting, either daily or living with the family.

National Curriculum
In 1988, the Government set down certain subjects that had to be learnt at school. In 1998, the core subjects are language and *literacy*, technology, science, human and social studies, mathematics, and physical education. Children are tested in these subjects at 7, 11 and 14, the key stages. Baseline testing is about to be introduced as children enter *infant school*.

National Society for the Prevention of Cruelty to Children (NSPCC)
A voluntary society that allows the public to report any cases of suspected *abuse* or *neglect*. In later years the society has become more active in preventing abuse and providing training.

natural immunity
Includes the body's natural defence mechanisms such as the skin, secretions and the *immune* system, the production of *antibodies* and *antitoxins* in response to

illness and the transfer of antibodies from the mother to the baby via the *placenta* and *breast-feeding*.

needs

All animals have primary needs, such as shelter and food. Human beings develop normally only when other needs are also met: security, *consistency of care* and affection with a sense of belonging to a group, and *cognitive* stimulation and *play*.

neglect

See *child protection*.

Neill, A.S. (1883–1973)

Scottish educationalist, who founded Summerhill School, a co-educational progressive school, free of authoritarian rules. He had some influence on 'progressive' education, his main philosophy being 'emotions are more important than intellect'. Introduced school councils, where the children made the rules.

neonate

A newborn infant: the first four weeks after birth.

nephritis

An inflammation of the kidney with a loss of *protein* and sometimes blood in the urine.

newborn

See *neonate*.

nodule

A small lump or swelling.

non-verbal communication

Sometimes called *body language*, where gestures and facial expressions convey quite clearly what the person is thinking, without the need to speak.

norm

Average performance, when a person's score on a test is compared with others. It is the standard expected.

nuclear family

A family composed of two parents and their children.

nursery class

These are attached to primary or *infant schools*, and most children in the class will go to the school when they are five. The staff ratio is 13 children to one staff (usually 26 children with a childcare practitioner and a teacher). There are advantages to being part of a school, sharing ancillary staff and other facilities. On the other hand, the outside play area is often more limited and, because there are less staff, it can be difficult for the children to benefit often from *one-to-one* attention.

nursery school

An educational establishment for children aged two to five years, either funded by the state, or private and fee-paying. State nursery schools offer a high standard of education and care, with a staff ratio of ten children to one staff. Usually, all the staff are trained, being either teachers or practitioners with the CACHE diploma or equivalent qualification. Private nursery schools vary more, some following the *Montessori* system whilst others may choose other programmes. To be a registered nursery, the private schools have to maintain good standards, but the quality of education may vary more than in the state system.

nutrition

The study of food and how it is used in the body.

O

obesity

Twenty per cent or more over ideal weight. More food is eaten than the body requires as energy and the excess is stored as fat. Often linked to lack of exercise.

object permanence

In *Piaget*'s terms, understanding that an object or a person does not cease to exist when out of sight.

objectivity

Making judgements from collected *data*, not allowing one's own feelings to be of any consequence.

observations

A close and careful examination and *monitoring* of individual children and children in groups. Childcare practitioners are the experts in carrying out observations of children using techniques such as *time* and *event samples, written records, flow charts, pie charts, bar charts, sociograms, histograms, longitudinal studies, child studies, target child studies*. They demonstrate objectively how children are achieving or behaving or reaching their developmental milestones.

obstetrics

A medical speciality concerned with women during pregnancy, childbirth and the recovery that follows. Childcare practitioners are occasionally employed on obstetric wards to support mothers with their new babies.

occupational therapy
The evaluation and treatment of physical and learning difficulties through activities and aids to enable people to function effectively in daily living.

oedema
Swelling of body tissue due to excess water content.

Oedipus complex
Oedipus was the King of Thebes who unknowingly killed his father and married his mother. The phrase, according to *Freud*, describes the feelings a son may have towards his father during the stage in his *emotional development* when he is strongly attached to his mother.

olfactory
Relating to smell.

oncology
The study of *tumours*.

one-to-one
An adult giving special attention to an individual child.

one-to-one correspondence
A mathematical term describing a developed concept of number, where a child matches one number to each object.

operant conditioning
A response continues to be made after being reinforced. For example, in *Pavlov*'s famous experiment with dogs, the dogs continued to salivate after the promise of a reward had been removed.

operational thinking
According to *Piaget*, the ability to logically manipulate signs and symbols.

ophthalmologist
A medically qualified specialist in diseases and disorders of the eye.

optic
Relating to the eye or vision.

oral
Relating to the mouth; **or** the tradition of storytelling.

oral stage
According to *Freud*, a child from birth to eighteen months seeks gratification by putting objects in his or her mouth – feeding being the most usual.

orchitis
Swollen and painful testicles often associated with *mumps*.

organised (ritual) abuse
Refers to *sexual abuse* and may involve *physical injury*. There will be a number of *perpetrators* and a number of abused children. There is an element of deliberate planning. It may refer to a *paedophile* ring, *prostitution*, or the involvement of children in the production of pornographic material.

organised games
When children reach the stage in their moral development when they can distinguish 'right' from 'wrong' they are able to take part in games that are structured and planned by adults, and *games with rules*.

organism
A living individual, which could be a single cell, or an individual plant or animal.

orthodontist
A dentist concerned mainly with the correction of misalignment and irregularities of the teeth.

orthopaedic medicine
Concentrates on conditions affecting muscles, joints, and bones.

orthoptist
A person qualified to detect and measure squints (*strabismus*) in children, to measure the visual acuity of each eye and to train the eye muscles.

ossification of bones
The process of change from soft cartilage and membrane to hard bone.

osteomyelitis
A *bacterial infection* of the bone.

otitis media
An *infection* of the middle ear that may be due to a *virus* or to *bacteria*.

outside play
All good pre-schools have an outside play area, and there should be free play inside and outside in most weathers, instead of just at prescribed times. Fresh air and *vigorous physical play* are good for the respiratory system, for the growth of large muscles, the encouragement of a good appetite and the prevention of *infection*.

oxytocin
A *hormone* that contracts the breast muscles, propelling milk to the nipple.

P

paediatrician
A doctor who specialises in diagnosing and treating children.

paedophile
An adult who preys on young children, with the aim of sexual assault.

palate
The roof of the mouth.

pallor
An abnormal lack of colour.

palmar grasp
Describes a primitive grasp, when the baby grabs objects with the whole hand.

pandemic
A worldwide *epidemic*.

parallel play
Playing alongside, but not necessarily with, another child.

paranoia
A mental disorder with delusions of persecution and self-importance.

parasites
Live on or in a living *organism*, deriving nourishment from the host. Examples of *infestation* in human beings are lice, fleas, *threadworms* and *scabies* mites.

parent and toddler groups
Similar to *drop in centres* in that the parents attend with their small children, but can be more formal, and usually charge a fee for attendance. A number of nursery classes and schools now operate parent and toddler groups.

Parent Teacher Associations (PTAs)
Associations formed so that teachers and parents can work together in partnership. PTAs are often involved in fund-raising.

parental involvement
Parents can be involved on a day-to-day basis, working in the classroom, in fund-raising, joining the *Parent Teacher Association*, helping on outings, helping with homework, becoming a parent governor, being on a management committee.

parental rights and responsibilities
Parents should have responsibility for their children, rather than rights over them. Parental responsibility is defined as the rights, duties, powers, responsibilities and authority that, by law, a parent of a child has in relation to the child and to his or her property (The *Children Act, 1989*).

paronychia
Infection of the nail bed.

partnership with parents
The *Children Act, 1989* has laid down firmly that parents have *rights and responsibilities*, and all professionals are expected to work with them in partnership for the benefit of the child.

passive immunity
Antibodies from an outside source given to the body, either naturally as in breast milk or via the *placenta*, or artificially in a *serum* containing antibodies produced by another person or animal.

pathogen
Any agent that can cause disease.

patterning
A *therapy* designed to improve the mobility of brain-injured children. A series of exercises that allow the undamaged part of the brain to take over the functions of the damaged part. Children are given intensive, frequent and repetitive rhythmic stimulation to their limbs.

Pavlov, Ivan (1849–1936)
Russian psychologist who based his work on the behaviour of dogs. Before they were fed, a bell was rung. Eventually, the dogs salivated at the ringing of the bell, without any food being offered. This is called classical conditioning.

pediculosis
Infestation with *lice*, named according to the body site. Pediculosis capitis refers to head lice.

peer
A member of one's age group.

peer group
People of the same age and stage.

peer pressure
The pressure exerted by groups to conform to the norms and values of the group.

percentile charts
Used to record the *growth* of children. Regular measurements of weight, length and *head circumference* are taken and plotted on the charts.

perception
An interpretation or impression based on personal understanding and past experiences.

perinatal mortality
Includes *stillbirth*s and deaths in the first week of life.

perineum
The tissue between the vagina and anus.

permanent teeth
The 32 teeth that start to appear from six years onwards.

perpetrator
The person responsible for an action. The term usually describes a person who is *abusing* children.

person specification
A detailed list setting out the qualifications, skills, knowledge and attitudes essential or desirable in anyone applying for a specific post.

personal development
This includes *aesthetic development*, *moral development*, *spiritual development*, and *creativity*.

personality
The distinctive characteristics or qualities of a person. *Jung* describes the introvert and the extrovert personality, the first type being reserved, and the second more outgoing.

perspiration
The act of sweating.

pertussis
Another name for *whooping cough*.

petit mal
A mild form of *epilepsy* with only a momentary loss of consciousness. See *absences*.

phallic stage
Time of the family romance, according to *Freud*'s *Oedipus complex* in boys, and Electra complex in girls around the ages of three to six years. Zone of gratification moves to the genital region.

phenylketonuria (PKU)
An inherited metabolic disorder, which prevents the normal digestion of *protein*. The child is unable to utilise the *amino acid* phenylalanine. If untreated, brain damage will occur. All children are screened within days of birth by a blood test (*Guthrie test*).

phobia
An irrational or unreasonable fear held by someone who is unable to control or dispel it.

phosphorus
An essential *mineral* that combines with *calcium* for strong bones and teeth.

photophobia
Sensitivity to light.

phototherapy
Exposure to ultraviolet rays for periods of time. Used for treating *jaundice* in the *neonate*.

physical abuse and injury
Intentional, non-accidental use of physical force and violence, resulting in hurting, injuring or destroying a child. It includes poisoning.

physical development
Describes how the body becomes more skilled and complex in its abilities. It will involve movement that is divided into *gross* and *fine motor development*.

physical neglect
A failure by parents/carers to provide adequately for the needs and safety of their children. It is not always intentional. Some parents/carers will put their own needs and interests first and neglect the child, while others might be unwell or unable to cope.

physiology
Knowledge and understanding of the function and processes of the body and its systems, what happens in the living body and how it happens.

physiotherapy
The treatment of disorders of movement and function in the body, caused by problems in the muscles, bones and nervous system. Treatment can involve exercise, manipulation, heat, and electrical or ultrasonic

procedures. The treatment is carried out by physiotherapists.

Piaget, Jean (1896–1980)

Swiss psychologist, best known for his research into intelligence, and the theory that a child will use inherited ability together with the *environment* to develop *cognitively* (nature plus nurture). Although he used a very small sample (his own children) Piaget was meticulous in his *observations* and *data* collecting. He showed that all children go through certain stages, and that these stages follow the same sequence: *sensori-motor, pre-operational, concrete operations,* and *formal operations*. Since the child's development results from exploring and interacting with the environment, the richer and more stimulating the environment, the more rapidly will a child develop. He has had a great influence on school systems since the 1960s

pica

To develop an abnormal appetite for eating earth, wood, paper, coal, etc. May be associated with *anaemia*, not resulting from worms, but worms may result from eating dirt. May be associated with *toxoplasmosis*.

pie charts

A round chart, divided up into different pieces, like a pie, that shows information graphically. Can be used in *observations*.

pincer grasp

Use of index finger and thumb to pick up objects.

pityriasis rosea

Thought to be caused by a *virus*. It is signalled by one patch, of a single round eruption, on the body (herald patch) one or two weeks before an extensive *rash* develops all over the body.

placebo

A harmless substance given in place of medicine.

placenta

A disc-shaped organ that develops in the *uterus* during pregnancy, linking the *fetus* with the mother via the umbilical cord.

placing reflex

If the front of a baby's leg is in contact with the edge of a table, the baby will raise a leg and take a 'step' up on to the table.

plans and routines

Refers to the planning of activities in the classroom, and the general routines undertaken with the children.

plaque (dental)

A thin deposit on the teeth, a mixture of *mucus*, *bacteria* and food.

play

Play can be social, when children interact with each other; some researchers look on play as a process of socialisation. Children's play also reflects *cognitive* ability and development and is often described as the 'work of childhood'. See *lap play, cradle play, solo play, parallel play, associative play,* and *co-operative play* (stages of play) and *imitative play, domestic play, role play, imaginative play, spontaneous play, structured play, vigorous physical play, outside play, creative play, symbolic play,* and *organised games* (types of play).

play therapy

A therapy using *play* and dolls, to help children with various disorders, and those who have been *abused*.

playbus

Buses that visit different areas, perhaps on crowded housing estates, or in rural areas, with toys and equipment on board to meet the needs of the children. Playbuses may be hired by organisations running conferences, and used as *crèches*.

playgroup

Playgroups (often known as pre-schools) contain a number of young children between the ages of two and five, often on a sessional basis, and usually have some parents on the management committee and/or helping out from time to time in the running of the group. These groups can be full-time, and are sometimes run by voluntary agencies such as Save the Children and Barnado's. They originated in the fifties and sixties, when there were fewer *nursery classes* and *nursery schools*, particularly in middle class areas where *pre-school provision* was deemed unnecessary. They started out as a social place for children to play and parents to meet, but have evolved into more educational provision. A small charge is made for each session. Training is offered by the Pre-school Learning Alliance (PLA: originally the Pre-school Playgroup Association, the PPA).

playschemes

Run for children during the school holidays, usually with one trained person and unqualified assistants. They help parents who need to work, and keep the children occupied for part of the holidays. They can be run by voluntary associations or by the local authority.

playwork
The involvement of adults who wish to help and support children's play in a variety of settings designed for children between the ages of five and fifteen to play within an environment dedicated to play.

playworker
In educational terms, the person who works, usually in a team of people, to provide *play* opportunities for children outside school hours and during the holidays.

pneumonia
An *infection* of the lung itself rather than just the air passages. It may be secondary to another problem such as *asthma* or it may follow another infection such as *measles*, it is then known as bronchopneumonia.

policies and procedures in child protection
These include *child protection conferences*, the *central register*, *child protection plans*, *child protection reviews* and *deregistration*.

policies and procedures in establishments
Procedures concerning children, such as exclusion, accidents, *child protection*, admissions, food, use of volunteers, bringing and collecting children, *partnership with parents*, outings, *assessment*, the *curriculum* and fire drill, and polices concerning staff, such as *appraisal*, *grievance procedures*, dismissal, *disciplinary procedures*, training and meetings.

polio vaccine
Given orally protects against *poliomyelitis*.

poliomyelitis
A *virus* that attacks the nervous system and can cause permanent muscle paralysis. It has been almost wiped out by routine *immunisation*.

Portage
An early learning resource for children with special needs providing a home-based daily teaching and learning programme.

positive affirmative action
The decision by an organisation to *discriminate* in favour of a disadvantaged group in order to improve their position.

positive images
Developing a positive *environment* that reflects all the children in a positive way, for example showing women carrying out what traditionally have been thought of as men's roles. It is against *stereotyping* by *race*, *gender* and *disability*. It should be reflected in books, posters, food, festivals and artefacts and in the involvement of all the parents.

positive reinforcement
Praise and other rewarding actions, endorsing an achievement or improvement in *behaviour*, with the expectation of positive continued change.

possetting
Regurgitation of a small amount of milk after the baby has been fed.

post-neonatal mortality
Deaths at 28 days and over up to one year.

post-term (post mature) baby
Born after 41 completed weeks of pregnancy.

posture
A position of the limbs or body.

potassium
A *mineral* that plays a part in maintaining fluid balance.

poverty
The lack of adequate resources to satisfy essential minimum human needs. It can be relative, being very poor in an affluent society, or absolute, being near to starvation.

precocity
Unusually early development of capabilities.

pre-conception
The time between deciding to have a baby and the time the baby is conceived.

pre-disposing factors of abuse
It is suggested that there are many factors, environmental, economic and psychological, that might provide sufficient stress to lead to *abuse* and/or *neglect*.

pre-eclampsia (toxaemia of pregnancy)
A complication in pregnancy, demonstrated by raised blood pressure, *protein* in the urine, swollen hands and feet, and sometimes excessive weight gain. If it is not controlled then eclampsia (toxaemia) will develop resulting in epileptic-type *convulsions*, with a very poor *prognosis* for the mother and baby,

prejudice
A set of beliefs, generally fixed, that is learned and leads to bias for or against a particular group or idea.

pre-operational stage
The second major stage of intellectual development, according to *Piaget*, when children (two- to seven-year-olds) are able to think in symbols but have not grasped logic.

prepuce
The foreskin of the penis.

pre-schools
See *playgroups*.

pre-school provision
Refers to the care and education provided for children under school age. It can be care in the home, by the parents, the extended family, a *nanny*, an *au pair*, a *mother's help* or a *child-minder*. It can be care in a *daycare establishment*. It can refer to care with a parent or carer present, such as a *toy library*, *special classes*, a *playbus*, a *drop in centre*, or a *parent and toddler group*. It also describes *crèches*, *playgroups* and *educational pre-school provision*, such as *nursery schools*, *nursery classes*, *special schools*, and *extended day provision*.

pre-term (premature) baby
Born before 37 weeks of pregnancy.

Primary Health Care (PHC) team
A *multi-disciplinary team*, usually working in a *health centre* or group practice, that includes doctors, *health visitors*, nurses, midwives, *social workers*, *dieticians*, physiotherapists (see *physiotherapy*), and speech therapists (see *speech therapy*).

primitive reflexes
Seen in the newborn baby such as *rooting*, *grasp*, *Moro*, *startle*, *placing* and *walking* reflexes. They disappear at different times but by three months they have been replaced by voluntary, learned responses.

private nurseries
Run for profit, but some have places for children who may need *daycare*, paid for by *social services*.

private provision
Educational and *daycare* provision that is paid for by the *customer*.

professional associations
Organisations that exist for people within certain professions, offering support and guidance. The Professional Association for Nursery Nurses (PANN) and the Professional Association for Teachers (PAT) differ from unions in that they undertake not to go on strike, but to seek negotiation by other means.

professional development
The continued updating of skills and knowledge that is necessary for successful good practice.

professional practice
Includes *teamwork*, *partnership with parents*, *professional associations* and *codes of practice*.

prognosis
Predicting the course and probable outcome of a disease.

prolactin
A *hormone* essential for the production of milk.

prone
Lying face down.

prophylaxis
The prevention of disease, or measures taken that are necessary to prevent disease.

prosthesis
The replacement of a missing or failing body part with an artificial substitute.

protect
See *child protection*.

protein
One of the main food groups. Made up of amino acids, protein is essential for *growth* and repair of all body tissues and helps to make *antibodies*.

protein food
Animal *proteins* alone supply all essential *amino acids*; vegetable and plant protein by themselves do not provide all amino acids. A good varied mixture is needed to supply complete requirements.

protozoa
Single cell animal *micro-organisms* that can cause diseases such as *dysentery* and *malaria*.

psoriasis
A chronic skin condition recognised by silvery grey scales covering red patches on the skin. It is not *contagious*.

psychiatrist
A medically qualified specialist in mental illness.

psychological factors of abuse
It can be the psychological make-up of one parent that leads to *abuse* or *neglect*.

psychologist
A person trained to assess *behaviour*al patterns, to measure *IQ* and assess development and to recognise *learning difficulties*.

psychology
Study of the *behaviour* of the individual.

public health
Measures to ensure the *health* of the general population including pure water, safe disposal of sewage and rubbish, controlling pollution, good housing, notification of disease, registration of births and deaths and burial of the dead.

puerperal psychosis
A very severe condition following childbirth where the mother undergoes a personality change and loses contact with reality. She is unable to function effectively or to relate to the baby or other people.

pyloric stenosis
Results from an overgrowth of the muscle surrounding the lower end of the stomach, when milk cannot leave the stomach and is vomited instead (projectile *vomiting*). It is resolved by surgery.

pyrexia
A raised body temperature resulting in fever.

Q

quarantine period
The time in which a person with a specific *infection* is capable of transferring that infection to other people.

R

race
Each of the major divisions of human kind, having distinct physical characteristics and connected by common descent.

race relations
Relationships between different races. The Race Relations Act makes it illegal to *discriminate* against another person because of his or her *race*.

racial harassment
Creating a hostile atmosphere for people of different *ethnic* groups by making derogatory remarks, negative statements, provocative *behaviour*, graffiti and racist jokes.

racism
Supports the idea of one superior *race* or *culture*.

rapid eye movement sleep
Occurs in the lighter stages of sleep when dreaming occurs, the eyes can be seen moving rapidly under the eyelids.

rash
A general term applied to any eruption of the skin.

recessive genes
Both parents have to be carriers of the defective *gene*. Each child has a one in four chance of having the condition. Each child will have a two in one chance of being a carrier for the condition, e.g. *cystic fibrosis*, *sickle cell*.

reconstituted family
Resulting from divorce, separation and re-marriage. The coming together of groups of children into *families* with new parents/carers.

record keeping
Keeping careful *written records* of the children's achievements is vital. Records should be kept in the *pre-school* and all through the school years. The parents have a right to see them, if they should so wish.

recovery position
Used by a first aider to position the body of an unconscious person who is still breathing. This position is comfortable, eases breathing, and prevents the tongue slipping back and blocking the airway.

references
A written or oral testimonial regarding character and capabilities, often requested prior to employment; **or** drawing attention to a piece of writing elsewhere.

referral
Arranging for a specialist doctor or an agency to see a child, generally for advice or treatment.

reflex
An involuntary reaction to stimuli.

register

A legal document used to record the attendance or non-attendance of the child in school or nursery; **or** to list persons 'fit' to work with children, and held by the local authority.

registration

Local authorities have a legal duty to keep a register of all child-minding and *daycare* provision and to ensure minimum standards of care. People on the register will be inspected at least once a year. See also *central register* and *registers*.

regressive behaviour

When a child is ill, or emotionally upset, his or her *behaviour* may be more suitable for someone younger. For example, a child who can normally concentrate well, finds it impossible to do more than play with toys and equipment that would normally be considered too young. He or she might start wetting the bed again, having been completely dry for more than a year.

relapse

To become ill again after an apparent recovery.

repetitive habits

Such as head banging, ear and hair pulling, tooth grinding, lip and tongue sucking. Generally indicate an emotional need.

repetitive play

Continually returning to one type of play. Although eventually the child should be encouraged to move on and try something else, it does help instil *learning* in the memory of the child.

residential care

Homes provided by the local authority, that care for children 'at risk' in one way or another. Known not to be an ideal form of care, many homes have closed, and most children are eventually placed with *foster* parents, or go back to their own *family*.

resources

In educational and *daycare* establishments resources refers to toys and equipment, staff and buildings. In a text book it refers to books, videos, useful addresses etc.

respite care

Short-term residential care for children with *disabilities*, to give the family a rest. Often used to assess the child's needs.

resuscitation

The restoration of respiration and circulation. It is a technique taught on first aid courses and essential knowledge for the childcare practitioner.

review of services

Each local authority, together with the local education authority, must carry out a three-year review of all *daycare* services and *supervised activities for children* under eight.

reviews

Regular meetings to reassess children on the *child protection register* and the *child protection plan*. The term is also used more generally, to meet to discuss children and staff progress etc.

rewards and punishments

Used to modify *behaviour*. For example, stars on a chart might encourage children in a school to work harder, or sweets can be given to reinforce good *behaviour*.

rhesus incompatibility

Occurs when a rhesus negative mother has her second or subsequent rhesus positive baby. The mother may have developed *antibodies* to the positive factor during her first pregnancy. All negative mothers are given an injection of Anti-D after the births of their babies to protect future babies.

rickets

A defective *growth* of bones due to *vitamin* D *deficiency*. It is rare these days but occasionally seen in children whose diet is inadequate and who have little exposure to the sun.

rights

The United Nations Convention on the Rights of the Child, adopted in 1989, set down the basic principles for the welfare and protection of children. It focuses the world's attention on the needs of children as it attempts to provide detailed minimum standards of care for all children.

ringworm

A *fungus infection* of different types that may affect the skin or nails. It produces circular *rashes*, which spread in ever increasing circles while healing in the centre. The active edge is raised into small bumps. On the scalp it will result in bald patches.

role model

A person looked to by others as an example in a particular situation. For example, a good teacher.

role play

Pretending to be mothers and fathers, superheroes and teachers allows children to *empower* themselves and find out about the real world. Role play is also used as a teaching aid, with students taking on the role of others, for example to feel what it might be like to be *disabled* or a small child.

roles

The parts that one plays during life. One person has many roles: for example, a woman might be a mother, a daughter, a grandmother, a sister, a doctor, a wife, a chairperson, a guide leader and so on during the same period. See *role play*.

rooting reflex

If one side of the baby's cheek or mouth is touched gently the head will turn in the direction of the touch.

rote learning

Learning by repetition, for example chanting 'times tables'.

routines, understanding and setting up

Regular activities organised and planned co-operatively and undertaken by everyone, such as hand-washing, eating, rest and sleep, exercise and play.

rubella (German measles)

An *infectious* disease caused by the rubella *virus*. It is a very mild disease in children but can cause damage to the *fetus* in the early stages of pregnancy.

S

safety checks

All equipment used in *pre-schools*, schools and nurseries needs to be checked frequently for any *hazard*.

saliva

Secretion of the salivary glands in the mouth, it is used to lubricate food and start the process of digestion.

salt

A *mineral* that helps to maintain the fluid balance of the body.

scabies

A skin *infestation* caused by the scabies mite.

scald

To burn with hot liquid or steam.

scapegoating

Blaming a person unfairly for the shortcomings or problems of others.

scarlet fever

An illness caused by *streptococcus bacteria* entering the body via the tonsils. It is less common and less dangerous than it once was.

schema

Refers to the basic *cognitive* unit, and consists of the perceiver's knowledge and beliefs about something.

schizophrenia

A psychotic or mental derangement.

scientific activities

Early scientific activities would include sorting, classifying and comparing, asking questions, investigating and observing. The scientific method can be instilled at an early age, by showing children how to observe, questioning what they see, investigating, and experimenting. Activities can be carried out which embrace most of these: cooking is one, gardening another.

scoliois

A twisting deformity of the spine so that there are curvatures from side to side.

screening

Simple tests which can detect early disease and abnormality, for example the *Guthrie test* for *phenylketonuria*, cervical screening and hearing tests.

seborrhoeic eczema

Seen in babies. Red inflamed patches on the skin creases of the groin, buttocks, behind the ear on the scalp and neck, and in the armpit. It is often associated with *cradle cap*.

seizure

See *convulsions*.

self-esteem

Confidence in oneself as a worthwhile person. Essential to *learning* and achievement. *Abused* children often suffer from low self-esteem.

self-reliance

Independence. From a very young age, children strive

to do things for themselves, such as dressing and washing. This can be helped by adult encouragement, which sometimes needs patience

senses
Vision, hearing, touch, smell and taste. Babies learn initially through all the senses.

sensori-motor stage
In *Piaget*'s terms, the first stage of development (birth to two years), when children gather information predominantly through their senses.

sensori-neural hearing impairment
Damage to the nervous system and the hearing mechanism, resulting from a variety of different causes such as viral *infections*, brain damage, maternal *rubella*, and *genetic* inheritance.

sensory impairment
When one of the senses is either damaged, or not fully developed.

separation anxiety
Felt by young children when taken away from their primary caregiver. A normal stage of development in 6-months to year old children.

sepsis
Infection.

septicaemia
Infection caused by *micro-organisms* in the blood.

serum
Blood plasma (fluid) from which the clotting factors have been removed. Serum is also used in *artificial passive immunity* when it may contain *antibodies* and *antitoxins* made by another human or animal and given by injection.

sessional care
Care offered for short, well defined periods of time, for example a pre school that might run from 9.30 to 11.30 am, close, and then run from 1.30 to 3.30 pm. Children may attend one or both sessions, but will not be cared for over the lunch period.

sex tourism
Some countries are known for providing children for sex for tourists. If the *perpetrators* are British they can now be taken to court in the UK.

sex-linked disorder
A *genetic* disorder carried by the female, but the condition is only seen in male children e.g. in

haemophilia, *Duchenne muscular dystrophy* and *colour vision defects*.

sexual abuse
The involvement of dependent, developmentally immature children or adolescents in sexual activities that they do not fully comprehend, to which they are unable to give informed consent, or that violate the social taboos of *family* roles. In other words, the use of children for sexual gratification (Schechter and Roberge, 1976). It can occur in any age group with both boys and girls by men and women.

sexual harassment
'Unwanted conduct of a sexual nature based on sex, affecting the dignity of women and men at work' (EU Code of Conduct).

sexual orientation
Human beings are usually attracted by the opposite sex (*heterosexuality*). Some people prefer to be intimate with people of the same sex (*homosexuality*), while others are attracted to both sexes (*bisexuality*).

sexually transmitted diseases (venereal diseases)
Any of various diseases such as gonorrhoea and syphilis that are transmitted by sexual contact or intercourse.

sibling
Brother or sister.

sibling rivalry
The *jealousy* that a child, or an adult, might feel towards his or her brother or sister.

sickle cell anaemia
A *chronic genetic* condition affecting children from birth. It is commonly found in people of Afro-Caribbean and African descent and is sometimes found in people from the Middle East, India and Pakistan. It is a blood disorder where abnormal haemoglobin is produced, assuming a sickle shape that is not fully oxygenated. It is an extremely painful distressing condition. *Genetic counselling* is available.

side effect
Any unwanted non-therapeutic effect caused by a drug or treatment. A generally undesirable secondary effect.

significant harm
The term used to decide whether the harm that has been done to the child from *abuse* or *neglect* will have

long-term effects on the development of the child. This *concept* is embodied within the *Children Act, 1989.*

signs of illness
Any observable evidence of a disease.

sinusitis
Infection in one or more of the air-filled cavities in the skull that link with the nose.

Skinner, Burrhus Frederick (1904–1990)
American behavioural psychologist, believed in nurture, not nature. Worked with rats that learnt how to press levers and pigeons that he taught to play ping-pong. The reward of food was a reinforcement, as the animals learnt that by carrying out the task they would be fed. This was called *operant conditioning* and most *behaviours* can be conditioned in this way. Led to the development of programmed learning and *behaviour modification.*

social and environmental factors of abuse
Takes place when the family is under stress for reasons of *poverty*, drug and alcohol abuse, divorce, unemployment, *reconstituted families*, and so on. If the stress becomes too much, this may lead to *abuse* or *neglect.*

social development
Learning to develop into a social being, at first in the *family* and then through the influence of *peers* and others in the outside world.

social model of disability
Suggests that society disables people by creating barriers, displaying *discrimination* and *prejudice.* The cure is to restructure *society.*

social security
Public provision for the economic welfare of certain groups such as the elderly and the unemployed, through pensions and other benefits.

social services departments
A department of the local authority which has responsibilities laid down by law to protect vulnerable groups of people and to provide services for them, generally the elderly, people with disabilities, and children. They have *statutory* functions under the *Children Act, 1989.*

social services provision of daycare
Usually provided for lone parents so that they can return to work, and is also provided for children thought to be at risk.

social workers
People employed by the local authority or *voluntary* organisations that work with many different *clients* and problems. They have many *statutory* responsibilities and should be able to cope with conflict and making difficult decisions. They may be involved in individual and *family* casework, group work and community work.

socialisation
The way the family initially, and later the outside *environment*, influences the child to act in an acceptable manner.

society
The customs and organisation of an ordered community. Society can be referred to as closed, as in a boarding school or a pre-literate society, where there is little contact with the outside world, or open where the society changes with the influences in the *environment.*

sociograms
Charts showing friendships. Can be used in *observations.*

solo play
Playing on one's own.

soundbeam
An adjustable, invisible soundbeam provides music which has a pleasurable and peaceful effect. For children with *special needs*, it can be operated by the slightest movement of a finger, hand or eye. Rocking in the beam can produce different sounds of varying tones and intensity.

soya milk
Milk produced from the *protein* of the soya bean and glucose.

spacer
Equipment used by children under five years with *asthma*. The medicine is puffed into the spacer at one end and then *inhaled* by the child via a mask at the other end. See *inhalers.*

spatial awareness
Learning to be aware and to control one's body in relation to space, other objects and people, so that children can move safely and with confidence.

special classes for pre-schoolers
Gym, music, dancing and creative art classes, among

others, are provided for the very young. Swimming is also popular, and there are special classes for babies.

special diets

Planned by the doctor and *dietician* according to the individual needs of the child, generally for specific conditions such as *obesity*, *failure to thrive*, *vitamin* and *mineral deficiency disorders*, *coeliac disease*, *cystic fibrosis*, *phenylketonuria*, and *diabetes mellitus*. The diet will be supervised regularly by the community or hospital *dietician*.

special needs

Refers to children with varied *disabilities* or gifts, who may need special education.

special schools

Schools for children with *disabilities*, involving a *multidisciplinary team* of teachers, childcare practitioners, therapists and special aides. There are fewer schools than previously, as current thinking is to integrate as many children with *disabilities* as possible in mainstream schools.

speech therapy

Aims to enable clients to maximise their *communication skills*. Speech therapists work with children who have difficulty with speech, understanding, spoken or written language, using language, eating or drinking, and also seek a cause for the indistinct speech.

spina bifida

The bony spine that helps to protect the spinal cord fails to develop properly prior to birth. The nerves are exposed and unprotected. In some children the defect is very mild but in others the loss of function in the lower part of the back is complete. It is associated with *hydrocephalus*.

spiritual development

Concerned with the soul or spirit as opposed to material things.

spontaneous play

Happens throughout life, when a child or an adult decides to take part in an unstructured and untimed activity, purely for enjoyment.

sputum

Spit and *mucus* secretions *coughed* up from the respiratory passages.

squint

See *strabismus*.

staffing ratios

The number of staff employed in relation to the number of children in any establishment. The *Children Act, 1989* gives guidance as to the minimum ratios; the local authority may impose higher requirements.

stages of play

Solo play, parallel play, associative play, co-operative play and *games with rules*.

Standard Assessment Tasks (SATs)

SATs are part of the *National Curriculum*, and test children's achievements at regular intervals throughout their school career.

staphylococci

Bacteria that cause the majority of *boils*, *abscesses* and superficial skin *infection*. They also cause *pneumonia*. They are constantly present on the skin and in the nose.

staple foods

Generally *carbohydrate*, commonly eaten and forming the bulk of a diet, e.g. bread, potatoes, rice, millet.

startle reflex

At a sudden loud noise the baby's arms will move outwards with the elbows bent and the hands closed.

state provision

Educational and *daycare* provision that is paid for and provided by the state.

statutory

Refers to organisations, provision, rights, benefits, grants, etc. required by law to be provided by the state.

Steiner, Rudolf (1861–1925)

An Austrian social philosopher who founded schools initially for children with emotional and *learning difficulties*, and believed in training the 'innate human capacity for *spiritual* perception'. There are many Steiner schools in existence.

stereotypes

Generalisations about a particular group in *society*, for example believing that girls read earlier than boys.

stereotyping

Conforming to an unjustifiable fixed mental picture of *disability*, of *race*, of *class*, or of men or women. A form of *prejudice*.

sterilisation of equipment

To destroy all *pathogenic organisms* and spores generally by the use of chemicals or boiling water.

stillbirth
A baby born dead after 24 weeks of pregnancy.

stimulation
A situation or action that requires a response that is necessary for normal development.

stool
Waste matter (faeces) evacuated from the bowel through the anus.

strabismus (squint)
A turning inwards or outwards of one eye. A child with this appears to be looking in different directions.

stranger anxiety
Babies may be disturbed when a person they do not know comes near to them, or they are taken to a strange place. Usually occurs between the ages of six months and fifteen months.

streptococci
Highly potent *bacteria* that cause a range of *infections* from *tonsillitis*, ear infections and sore throats to *pneumonia* and *septicaemia*.

structured play
Prepared and planned carefully by the staff team, to develop particular areas of children's development.

subdural haematoma
A swelling containing blood between the outer and middle layers of the membranes that cover the brain. It may be caused by birth *trauma*, accidents, *meningitis*, or *child abuse*.

subjectivity
Dealing with matters in a personal way.

sudden infant death syndrome (SIDS)
The unexpected, unexplained and sudden death of an infant. A great deal has been learnt recently about the factors that might cause this, and includes parents who smoke and the position in which the baby is placed for sleep. This is sometimes referred to as 'cot death'.

suffocation
To deprive of oxygen by obstruction of the air passages.

supervision of children
Children need to be closely watched for their own safety, particularly when in the *outside play* area, using potentially dangerous tools, near water, or on outings.

supervisor
Students will have a person in their placements, usually a trained childcare practitioner, who will help them to progress, sort out any problems, and assess their competence.

supine
Lying on the back.

surma
Asian eye cosmetic that can contain lead.

surveillance
To watch over. Describes *assessment* programmes for selected age groups, for example monitoring developmental progress; **or** can be used by parents to monitor employees.

SWOT analysis
An exercise used by management to look at a proposed change or expenditure. To look at **S**trengths and **W**eaknesses of the organisation and compare with the **O**pportunities and **T**hreats from outside. It may be adapted and used in other circumstances.

symbolic play
A child uses an object to represent something else, for example, a child might use a brick and pretend it is a car.

symmetrical
Balanced movements of both sides of the body.

symptoms of illness
Any *subjective* change from the normal experienced by the patient that indicates an illness.

syndrome
A group of signs and symptoms that occur together and are characteristic of a disease or condition.

T

tactile
Connected with touch.

talipes (clubfeet)
Deformity of the ankle and foot, seen at birth, where the foot is bent either inwards or outwards.

tantrum
Violent display of uncontrollable rage.

target child
A form of *observation* devised by Kathy Sylva, that is used as a tool to study concentration in *pre-school* children.

teamwork
A group of people working together with common and well understood aims and objectives, having the ability to be flexible and to *communicate* well.

teeth types
Incisor, canine, premolar and molar.

tepid sponging
Using lukewarm water to slowly reduce a raised body temperature.

term baby
A baby born between 37 and 41 completed weeks of pregnancy.

terminal illness
Incurable illness, leading to death. Patients are often cared for in *hospices* or nursed at home.

terminology
The correct terms used in a particular subject.

test weighing
A method of assessing how much milk a breast-fed baby consumes over a 24 hour period. The baby is weighed immediately before a feed and then again after the feed, before the napkin is changed. The difference is recorded and all the feeds are added up over the 24 hours.

testes
Male sex organs.

tetanus (lockjaw)
Occurs when *toxins* of the tetanus *bacteria* affect the central nervous system. It is prevented by *immunisation*.

thalassaemia
A generic term for a number of *genetic* blood disorders in which there is insufficient haemoglobin. It is found in children from southern Mediterranean countries and the Middle East. *Genetic counselling* is available.

themes and topics
Used by teachers and childcare practitioners to bring about '*desirable outcomes*' (as required by the *National Curriculum*). For example, a topic might be 'transport'.

theories
Attempts to organise information in order to explain why certain events occur. The goal of a theory is to integrate *data* (or information), explain *behaviour* and predict behaviour.

therapy
A technical term for the treatment of diseases and disorders without the use of surgery.

thought
The process or power of thinking, the faculty of reason. Descartes stated 'I think, therefore I am'.

threadworms
Parasitic worms that live in the large bowel. They look like threads of cotton and may be seen round the anus or in the *stool*. They may be asymptomatic or cause irritation round the anus. This may result in *enuresis* or problems caused by lack of sleep.

thrush
Caused by a *fungus infection* called Candida albicans, resulting in white patches on the tongue and palate. It is very painful, and may interfere with feeding. It may also be seen in the napkin area.

thyroid deficiency (hypothyroidism)
Under-secretion of thyroxine from the thyroid gland. If untreated it slows down normal *growth* and development.

Thyroid Stimulating Hormone test (TSH)
A blood test to diagnose *hypothyroidism* taken at the same time as the *Guthrie test*.

tics
Habit spasms. Regular nervous habits such as twitching the nose, blinking, sniffing etc.

time sample
A sample of time when you observe a child over a fairly long period at fixed intervals. Particularly useful technique for studying withdrawn, sad and shy children, and those who find it difficult to make relationships.

toilet training
Encouraging children to achieve control of the bowel and bladder. This can not be attained until the central nervous system is sufficiently mature.

tonic/clonic seizure (grand mal)
A major *epileptic* fit, with loss of consciousness,

shaking, clenched teeth, and perhaps frothing at the mouth. The child will fall down and may pass urine. During the clonic phase the child may twitch.

tonsillitis
Infection of the lymphoid tissue at the back of the throat.

toxicariasis
The *infection* of humans with a type of roundworm found in dogs and cats.

toxin
Any of various poisonous substances produced by *micro-organisms* that stimulate the production of *antitoxins* in the body.

toxoid
A *toxin* that has been treated to reduce its toxicity and is used in *immunisation* to stimulate production of *antitoxins*.

toxoplasmosis
A parasitic condition in cats that can be passed on to humans. In preganancy, the *fetus* can be blinded or brain-damaged by the *virus*.

toy library
Provided by the local authorities for young children and for children with *special needs*. Toys can be borrowed free. The toys are usually sturdy and may be too expensive for some *families* to afford. They are often 'educational', and give the children a preview of some of the equipment they may find when they start school.

transitional object
An object, often a blanket or a soft toy, which a child carries around as a comforter, and usually takes to bed with him or her. It may be used until it disintegrates. Sometimes called a comfort object.

transmission of disease
Micro-organisms are spread from person to person in a number of ways: for example by droplet *infection*, when the spray sneezed or *coughed* into the air is *inhaled* by another person; through direct contact when touching the infected person; and indirect contact through *fomites*. Contaminated food and drink, *vectors*, *carriers*, inadequate *sterilisation* techniques, dirty needles and exposure to dust, earth and dirt where some *micro-organisms* can lie dormant for long periods of time can also transmit disease.

trauma
Any injury or wound to the body; **or** a powerful shock that may have long lasting effects.

travelling families
Do not live at a permanent address but move around the country often living a nomadic existence. The term includes gypsies who are a distinct racial group. Some travellers will settle for the winter months and move on for the summer. Their lifestyle restricts their access to *health* and *education services*, and exposes them to *stereotyping* and *discrimination*.

tremor
An involuntary fine quivering movement most easily seen in the hands.

tripod grasp
Use of thumb and first two fingers to pick up objects.

tuberculosis
An *infectious* disease caused by the tubercle *bacteria*, it is less common because of extensive *immunisation*.

tumour
Any abnormal swellings: a mass of tissue formed by a new growth of cells.

twins
Identical (uniovular or monozygotic) twins occur when one fertilised egg divides into two and each half is a separate baby; **or** non-identical (binovular, dizygotic) twins occur when two eggs are produced at ovulation and both are fertilised.

U

ulcer
An open sore or cut of the skin or mucous membranes.

ultrasound scan
A medical procedure to visualise internal body structures.

umbilicus
The navel or 'belly button'.

urticaria (nettle rash or hives)
A blotchy red swelling of the skin caused by the release of histamine in the affected areas. It is usually part of an *allergic* reaction.

uterus (womb)
A hollow pear shaped body organ used for implantation, carrying, and nourishing the *fetus* during pregnancy.

V

vaccination
Giving a *vaccine* either orally or by injection. Commonly known as *immunisation*.

vaccine
Solution containing a killed or altered strain of a *pathogenic micro-organism* given to allow the body to develop resistance to the disease.

vacuum extraction
A metal or rubber cap is placed on the baby's head and attached to a suction pump. The baby is then born by gentle traction.

value judgement
A *subjective* opinion.

values
The code of ethics (principles and beliefs) of a particular *culture* or of an individual that determines the way they live their lives.

vector
An *organism* that carries and transmits *infection* from one host to another such as an animal that carries the rabies *virus*.

vegan
A person who does not eat or use any animal products.

vegetarian
A person who excludes meat and fish and sometimes egg, milk and cheese, from the diet.

ventral suspension
The baby held in the air with the face down.

verification
Establishing the truth or correctness of an action or a piece of work. Used in colleges to confirm that the marking of the first marker is fair and consistent.

vernix caseosa
A white greasy substance that protects the skin of the *fetus* from its watery *environment* in the *uterus*.

verrucae (plantar *warts*)
Harmless growths on the skin of the foot that may become painful due to pressure of walking.

vertebra
The backbone.

vertical grouping
Sometimes called family grouping, it refers to children of different ages being in the same class. This is quite usual with the two-, three- and four-year olds in nursery schools and classes, and sometimes occurs in infant and primary schools. This type of grouping is common in small schools, particularly in rural areas.

viable
Capable of surviving. Is often used in relation to the *fetus* as viable outside the *uterus*.

vigorous physical play
Usually takes place outside, involving the use of large climbing equipment and wheeled toys. *Vigorous exercise* helps children's respiration and encourages and extends large muscle development and *gross motor* skills.

virus
Single cell *micro-organisms*, smaller than *bacteria* that can be seen with an electron microscope. *Antibiotics* are not effective against viruses.

visual discrimination
The ability to discern different shapes and colours. Good visual discrimination aids reading ability.

visual
Refers to sight and seeing.

vital signs
Signs of life: respiration, pulse, blood pressure, and temperature.

vitamins
Small organic substances found in plants and animals. The body needs small amounts but they are essential for health. Only vitamins D and K are made in the body. Vitamins A, D, E and K are fat-soluble and can be stored in the body. Vitamins B group and C are water-soluble and not stored in the body.

vocal
Refers to the individual making sounds.

voluntary nurseries
Usually started in socially deprived areas and run by

organisations and charities such as 'Save the Children and Barnado's. May be full- or part-time.

voluntary provision
Refers to organisations and provision that are started by charitable groups or communities. Usually they are part-funded by the state, having shown they are needed and wanted by the community.

vomiting
The violent expulsion of stomach contents.

Vygotsky, Lev (1896–1934)
Russian psychologist, interested in *cognitive* development and the relationship between language and thinking.

W

walking reflex
A baby held upright with the soles of the feet on a flat surface, and moved forward slowly will respond with 'walking steps'.

warts
Growths on the skin, mainly the hands, face or feet, caused by a *virus infection*.

Watson, John B. (1878–1958)
An American psychologist who has been called 'the father of modern behaviourism'. He believed that all humans could be trained, and tried to prove this by training a baby (little Albert) into fearing the soft toys he had always loved.

weal
A slightly raised area of skin, usually accompanied by intense itching.

weaning
The introduction of solid foods after *breast-* or *bottle-feeding*.

whey
The watery liquid that separates from the *curd* when milk is clotted.

whooping cough (*pertussis*)
An infectious disease caused by *bacteria* called Bordetella pertussis. It mainly affects the respiratory system; there is a characteristic *cough*. *Immunisation* is available.

withdrawn behaviour
Describes behaviour that includes *crying*, inability to make relationships, passivity and shyness, and a refusal to *communicate*.

working with parents
See *partnership with parents*.

workplace nurseries
Daycare provided by employers. By looking after the children of the workforce, workplace nurseries enable the parents to continue their careers.

written records
When carrying out *observations*, this is the commonest technique used to record a naturally occurring event or a structured activity.

Z

Zen macrobiotic diet
Based on unrefined cereals often excluding fruit and vegetables. Fluid intake is also restricted.

A

ACE	Advisory Centre for Education
ACPC	Area Child Protection Committee
ADCE	Advanced Diploma in Childcare and Education
ADHD	attention deficit hyperactivity disorder
AID	artificial insemination by donor
AIDS	acquired immune deficiency syndrome
ASBAH	Association for Spina Bifida and Hydrocephalus

B

BAAF	British Agencies for Adoption and Fostering
BAECE	British Association for Early Childhood Education
BCG	bacille Calmette-Guerin
BIBIC	British Institute for Brain Injured Children
BSE	bovine spongiform encephalitis
BSI	British Standards Institute
BSL	British Sign Language
BTEC	Business and Technology Education Council

C

CAB	Citizen's Advice Bureau
CACHE	Council for Awards in Children's Care and Education
CAO	Child Assessment Order
CAPT	Child Accident Prevention Trust
CASE	Campaign for State Education
CCE	Certificate in Childcare and Education
CCETSW	Central Council for Education and Training in Social Work
CDH	congenital dislocation of hip
CLEAR	Campaign for Lead Free Air
COMA	Committee on Medical Aspects of food policy
CP	cerebral palsy
CPAG	Child Poverty Action Group
CPR	Child Protection Register
CRE	Committee for Racial Equality
CSA	child sexual abuse
CSF	cerebrospinal fluid
CSIE	Centre for Studies in Inclusive Education
CVS	chorionic villus sampling
cv	curriculum vitae
CWAC	Children with Aids Charity

D

DfEE	Department for Education and Employment
DHA	District Health Authority
DHS	District Health Service
DNA	deoxyribonucleic acid
DNN	Diploma in Nursery Nursing
DoH	Department of Health
DPT	diphtheria, pertussis and tetanus triple immunisation
DRV	Dietary Reference Values
DSS	Department of Social Security
DTP	desktop publishing

E

EARs	Estimated Average Requirements
EBM	expressed breast milk
EDD	expected date of delivery
EEG	electroencephalogram
EHD	Environmental Health Department
EHV	Educational Home Visitor
EOC	Equal Opportunities Commission
EPO	Emergency Protection Order
EPOCH	End Physical Punishment of Children
ESL	English as a Second Language
ESR	erythocyte sedimentation rate
EU	European Union
EWO	Educational Welfare Officer
EYDP	Early Years Development Plan
EYTARN	Early Years Trainers Anti-Racist Network

F

FAS	fetal alcohol syndrome
FHSA	Family Health Service Authority
FIS	Family Income Support
FPA	Family Planning Association
FRES	Federation of Recruitment and Employment Services
FSID	Foundation for the Study of Infant Deaths
FWA	Family Welfare Association

G

GMS	Grant Maintained Status
GNVQ	General National Vocational Qualification
GP	General Practitioner

H

HAPA	Handicapped Adventure Playground Association
Hb	haemoglobin
HCG	human chorionic gonadotrophin
HiB	Haemophilus influenzae type B
HIV	human immunodeficiency virus
HMSO	Her Majesty's Stationery Office
HRT	hormone replacement therapy
HV	Health Visitor
HVA	Health Visitor Association

I

IEP	Individual Educational Plan
INSET	In Service Training
IQ	intelligence quotient
IUCD	intrauterine contraceptive device
IVF	*in vitro* fertilisation

K

KCN	Kids' Club Network

L

LAD	language acquisition device
LAN	Local Area Networks
LEA	Local Education Authority
LMS	local management of schools

M

MAMA	Meet A Mum Association
MENCAP	Royal Society for Mentally Handicapped Children and Adults
MIND	National Association for Mental Health
MMR	measles, mumps and rubella immunisation
MP	Member of Parliament

N

NACNE	National Advisory Committee on Nutrition Education
NAI	non-accidental injury
NAMCW	National Association for Maternal and Child Welfare
NANN	National Association of Nursery Nurses
NCB	National Children's Bureau
NCH	National Children's Home
NCMA	National Child-minding Association
NCNE	National Campaign for Nursery Education
NCT	National Childbirth Trust
NHS	National Health Service
NSPCC	National Society for the Prevention of Cruelty to Children
NTLA	National Toy Libraries Association
NTO	National Training Organisation
NVQ	National Vocational Qualification

O

OFSTED	Office for Standards in Education
OPCS	Office of Population Censuses and Surveys

P

PANN	Professional Association of Nursery Nurses
PC	personal computer
PC	politically correct
PER	Practice Evidence Record
PKU	phenylketonuria
PLA	Pre-school Learning Alliance
PMS	pre-menstrual syndrome
PPA	Pre-school Playgroup Association (now PLA)

Q

QCA	Qualifications and Curriculum Authority

R

RAM	random-access memory
REM	rapid eye movement
Rh	rhesus factor

RNIB	Royal National Institute for the Blind
RoSPA	Royal Society for the Prevention of Accidents

S

SAFP	serum alpha-fetoprotein
SATs	Standard Assessment Tasks
SCAA	Schools Curriculum and Assessment Authority
SCBU	Special Care Baby Unit
SCOPE	Cerebral Palsy Society
SEN	Special Educational Needs
SENCO	Special Educational Needs Co-ordinator
SENSE	National Deaf, Blind and Rubella Association
SIDS	sudden infant death syndrome
SMP	Statutory Maternity Pay
SSD	Social Services Department
STA	Specialist Teacher Assistant
STD	sexually transmitted diseases
StD	Standard Deviation
SW	Social Worker

T

TAMBA	Twins and Multiple Births Association

TB	tuberculosis
TEC	Training and Enterprise Council
TENS	transcutaneous nerve stimulation
TES	Times Educational Supplement
tlc	tender loving care
TSH	Thyroid Stimulating Hormone test

U

UAR	Unit Assessment Record
UN	United Nations
UNICEF	United Nations International Children's Emergency Fund.
URTI	upper respiratory tract infection
UTI	urinary tract infection
UK	United Kingdom

V

VDU	visual display unit

W

WAN	wide area network
WHO	World Health Organisation
www	world wide web

APPENDIX A: DEVELOPMENTAL NORMS

0 to 1 year

	Physical development – gross motor	Physical development – fine motor	Social and emotional development	Cognitive and language development
At birth	Reflexes: ■ Rooting, sucking and swallowing reflex ■ Grasp reflex ■ Walking reflex ■ Moro reflex If pulled to sit, head falls backwards If held in sitting position, head falls forward, and back is curved In supine (laying on back), limbs are bent In prone (laying on front), lies in fetal position with knees tucked up. Unable to raise head or stretch limbs	Reflexes: ■ Pupils reacting to light ■ Opens eyes when held upright ■ Blinks or opens eyes wide to sudden sound ■ Startle reaction to sudden sound ■ Closing eyes to sudden bright light	Bonding/attachment	Cries vigorously, with some variation in pitch and duration
1 month	In prone, lifts chin In supine, head moves to one side Arm and leg extended on face side Begins to flex upper and lower limbs	Hands fisted Eyes move to dangling objects	Watches mother's face with increasingly alert facial expression Fleeting smile – may be wind Stops crying when picked up	Cries become more differentiated to indicate needs Stops and attends to voice, rattle and bell
3 months	Held sitting, head straight back and neck firm. Lower back still weak When lying, pelvis is flat	Grasps an object when placed in hand Turns head right round to look at objects Eye contact firmly established	Reacts with pleasure to familiar situations/routines	Regards hands with interest Beginning to vocalise

continued

0 to 1 year continued

	Physical development – gross motor	Physical development – fine motor	Social and emotional development	Cognitive and language development
6 months	In supine, can lift head and shoulders In prone, can raise up on hands Sits with support Kicks strongly May roll over When held, enjoys standing and jumping	Has learned to grasp objects and passes toys from hand to hand Visual sense well established	Takes everything to mouth Responds to different emotional tones of chief caregiver	Finds feet interesting Vocalises tunefully Laughs in play Screams with annoyance Understands purpose of rattle
9 months	Sits unsupported Begins to crawl Pulls to stand, falls back with bump	Visually attentive Grasps with thumb and index finger Releases toy by dropping Looks for fallen objects Beginning to finger-feed Holds bottle or cup	Plays peek-a-boo – can start earlier Imitates hand-clapping Clings to familiar adults, reluctant to go to strangers – from about 7 months	Watches activities of others with interest Vocalises to attract attention Beginning to babble Finds partially hidden toy Shows an interest in picture books Knows own name
1 year	Walks holding one hand, may walk alone Bends down and picks up objects Pulls to stand and sits deliberately	Picks up small objects Fine pincer grip Points at objects Holds spoon	Cooperates in dressing Demonstrates affection Participates in nursery rhymes Waves bye-bye	Uses jargon Responds to simple instructions and understands several words Puts wooden cubes in and out of cup or box

1 to 4 years

	Physical development – gross motor	Physical development – fine motor	Social and emotional development	Cognitive and language development
1 year	Walks holding one hand, may walk alone Bends down and picks up objects Pulls to stand and sits deliberately	Picks up small objects Fine pincer grip Points at objects Holds spoon	Cooperates in dressing Demonstrates affection Participates in nursery rhymes Waves bye-bye	Uses jargon Responds to simple instructions and understands several words Puts wooden cubes in and out of cup or box
15 months	Walking usually well established Can crawl up stairs frontwards and down stairs backwards Kneels unaided Balance poor, falls heavily	Holds crayon with palmar grasp Precise pincer grasp, both hands Builds tower of 2 cubes Can place objects precisely Uses spoon which sometimes rotates Turns pages of picture book	Indicates wet or soiled pants Helps with dressing Emotionally dependent on familiar adult	Jabbers loudly and freely, with 2–6 recognisable words, and can communicate needs Intensely curious Reproduces lines drawn by adult
18 months	Climbs up and down stairs with hand held Runs carefully Pushes, pulls and carries large toys Backs into small chair Can squat to pick up toys	Builds tower of 3 cubes Scribbles to and fro spontaneously Begins to show preference for one hand Drinks without spilling	Tries to sing Imitates domestic activities Bowel control sometimes attained Alternates between clinging and resistance Plays contentedly alone near familiar adult	Enjoys simple picture books, recognising some characters Jabbering established 6–20 recognisable words May use echolalia (repeating adult's last word, or last word of rhyme) Is able to show several parts of the body, when asked Explores environment energetically
2 years	Runs with confidence, avoiding obstacles Walks up and down stairs both feet to each step, holding wall Squats with ease. Rises without using hands Can climb up on furniture and get down again Steers tricycle pushing along with feet Throws small ball overarm, and kicks large ball	Turns picture book pages one at a time Builds tower of 6 cubes Holds pencil with first 2 fingers and thumb near to point	Competently spoon feeds and drinks from cup Is aware of physical needs Can put on shoes and hat Keenly interested in outside environment – unaware of dangers Demands chief caregiver's attention and often clings Parallel play Throws tantrums if frustrated	Identifies photographs of familiar adults Identifies small-world toys Recognises tiny details in pictures Uses own name to refer to self Speaks in 2- and 3-word sentences, and can sustain short conversations Asks for names and labels Talks to self continuously

continued

1 to 4 years continued

	Physical development – gross motor	Physical development – fine motor	Social and emotional development	Cognitive and language development
3 years	Competent locomotive skills Can jump off lower steps Still uses 2 feet to a step coming down stairs Pedals and steers tricycle	Cuts paper with scissors Builds a tower of 9 cubes and a bridge with 3 cubes Good pencil control Can thread 3 large beads on a string	Uses spoon and fork Increased independence in self-care Dry day and night Affectionate and cooperative Plays cooperatively, particularly domestic play Tries to please	Can copy a circle and some letters Can draw a person with a head and 2 other parts of the body May name colours and match 3 primary colours Speech and comprehension well established Some immature pronunciations and unconventional grammatical forms Asks questions constantly Can give full name, gender and age Relates present activities and past experiences Increasing interest in words and numbers
4 years	All motor muscles well controlled Can turn sharp corners when running Hops on favoured foot Balances for 3–5 seconds Increasing skill at ball games Sits with knees crossed	Builds a tower of 10 cubes Uses 6 cubes to build 3 steps, when shown	Boasts and is bossy Sense of humour developing Cheeky, answers back Wants to be independent Plans games cooperatively Argues with other children but learning to share	Draws person with head, legs and trunk Draws recognisable house Uses correct grammar most of the time Most pronunciations mature Asks meanings of words Enjoys verses and jokes, and may use swear words Counts up to 20 Imaginative play well developed

4 to 7 years

	Physical development – gross motor	Physical development – fine motor	Social and emotional development	Cognitive and language development
4 years	All motor muscles well controlled Can turn sharp corners when running Hops on favoured foot Balances for 3–5 seconds Increasing skill at ball games Sits with knees crossed	Builds a tower of 10 cubes uses 6 cubes to build 3 steps, when shown	Boasts and is bossy Sense of humour developing Cheeky, answers back Wants to be independent Plans games cooperatively Argues with other children but learning to share	Draws person with head, legs and trunk Draws recognisable house Uses correct grammar most of the time Most pronunciations mature Asks meanings of words Enjoys verses and jokes, and may use swear words Counts up to 20 Imaginative play well developed
5 years	Can touch toes keeping legs straight Hops on either foot Skips Runs on toes Ball skills developing well Can walk along a thin line	Threads needle and sews Builds steps with 3–4 cubes Colours pictures carefully Can copy adult writing	Copes well with daily personal needs Chooses own friends Well-balanced and sociable Sense of fair play and understanding of rules developing Shows caring attitudes towards others	Matches most colours Copies square, triangle and several letters, writing some unprompted Writes name Draws a detailed person Speaks correctly and fluently Knows home address Able and willing to complete projects Understands numbers using concrete objects Imaginary play now involves make-believe games

continued

4 to 7 years continued

	Physical development – gross motor	Physical development – fine motor	Social and emotional development	Cognitive and language development
6 years	Jumps over rope 25 cm high Learning to skip with rope	Ties own shoe laces	Eager for fresh experiences More demanding and stubborn, less sociable Joining a 'gang' may be important May be quarrelsome with friends Needs to succeed as failing too often leads to poor self-esteem	Reading skills developing well Drawings more precise and detailed Figure may be drawn in profile Can describe how one object differs from another Mathematical skills developing, may use symbols instead of concrete objects May write independently
7 years	Rides a 2-wheel bicycle Improved balance	Skills constantly improving More dexterity and precision in all areas	Special friend at school Peer approval becoming important Likes to spend some time alone Enjoys TV and books May be moody May attempt tasks too complex to complete	Moving towards abstract thought Able to read Can give opposite meanings Able to write a paragraph independently

APPENDIX B: SEQUENCE OF LANGUAGE DEVELOPMENT

Children's language develops through a series of identifiable stages. These stages are sequential, as outlined below. The level of children's development depends partly on their chronological age, but their experience of language from an early age is, however, just as important a factor. If children are exposed to a rich language environment this will be reflected in their language development. Children who have not had this opportunity will not have had the same chances for development. It is important to take this into account when assessing a child's stage of language development.

Children who are bilingual may develop their languages at a slightly slower rate than children who are monolingual. This is to be expected as they have much more to learn. Given an environment that promotes language development, bilingual children will become proficient in both languages.

Approximate age	Developmental level
Birth	Involuntary cry
2–3 weeks	Signs of intentional communication: eye contact
4 weeks onwards	Cries are becoming voluntary, indicating for example, unhappiness, tiredness, loneliness Children may respond by moving their eyes or head towards the speaker, kicking or stopping crying
6 weeks onwards	Children may smile when spoken to Cooing and gurgling begin in response to parent's or carer's presence and voice, also to show contentment
1–2 months	Children may move their eyes or head towards the direction of the sound
3 months	Children will raise their head when sounds attract their attention
4 months	Playful sounds appear: cooing, gurgling, laughing, chuckling, squealing; these are in response to the human voice and to show contentment Children respond to familiar sounds by turning their head, kicking or stopping crying Shouts to attract attention

Approximate age	Developmental level
6 months	The beginning of babbling: regular, repeated sounds, e.g. *gegegegeg*, *mamamam*, *dadada*; children play around with these sounds. This is important for practising sound-producing mechanisms necessary for later speech Cooing, laughing and gurgling become stronger Children begin to understand emotion in the parent or carer's voice Children begin to enjoy music and rhymes, particularly if accompanied by actions
9 months	Babbling continues and the repertoire increases Children begin to recognise their own name May understand simple, single words, e.g. *No, Bye-bye* Children continue to enjoy music and rhymes and will now attempt to join in with the actions, e.g. playing pat-a-cake
9–12 months	Babbling begins to reflect the intonation of speech Children may imitate simple words. This is usually an extension of babbling, e.g. *dada* Pointing begins. This is often accompanied by a sound or the beginnings of a word. This demonstrates an increasing awareness that words are associated with people and objects
12 months	Children's vocabulary starts to develop. First word(s) appear, usually names of people and objects that the child is familiar with. They are built around the child's babbling sound repertoire Children understand far more than they can say. This is called a passive vocabulary They begin to be able to respond to simple instructions, e.g. 'Give me the ball', 'Come here', 'Clap your hands'
15 months	Active vocabulary development remains quite limited as children concentrate on achieving mobility Passive vocabulary increases rapidly Pointing accompanied by a single word is the basis of communication
18 months	Children's active vocabulary increases; this tends to be names of familiar things and people Children use their language to name belongings and point out named objects Generalisation of words is difficult, e.g. cat can only be their cat, not the one next door One word and intonation is used to indicate meaning, e.g. cup may mean, 'I want a drink', 'I have lost my cup', 'Where is my cup?'. The intonation (and possibly the situation) would indicate the meaning to people who are familiar with the child Children will repeat words and sentences

Approximate age	Developmental level
21 months	Both passive and active vocabularies rapidly increase; the passive vocabulary, however, remains larger than the active Children begin to name objects and people that are not there: this shows an awareness of what language is for Sentences begin. Initially as two word phrases, e.g. 'Mummy gone', 'Coat on' Gesture is still a fundamental part of communication Children begin asking questions, usually 'What?', 'Who?' and 'Where?'
2 years	Both active and passive vocabularies continue to increase Children can generalise words but this sometimes means that they over-generalise, e.g. all men are *daddy*, all furry animals with four legs are *dog* Personal pronouns (words used instead of actual names) are used, e.g. I, she, he, you, they. They are not always used correctly Sentences become longer although they tend to be in telegraphic speech, i.e. only the main sense-conveying words are used, e.g. 'Mummy gone work', 'Me go bike' Questions are asked frequently, 'What?' and 'Why?'
2 years 6 months	Vocabulary increases rapidly; there is less imbalance between passive and active vocabularies Word use is more specific so there are fewer over- and under-generalisations Sentences get longer and more precise, although they are still usually abbreviated versions of adult sentences Word order in sentences is sometimes incorrect Children can use language to protect their own rights and interests and to maintain their own comfort and pleasure, e.g. 'It's mine', 'Get off', 'I'm playing with that' Children can listen to stories and are interested in them
3 years	Vocabulary develops rapidly; new words are picked up quickly Sentences continue to become longer and more like adult speech Children talk to themselves during play: this is to plan and order their play, which is evidence of children using language to think Language can now be used to report on what is happening, to direct their own and others' actions, to express ideas and to initiate and maintain friendships Pronouns are usually used correctly Questions such as 'Why?', 'Who?' and 'What for?' are used frequently Rhymes and melody are attractive

Approximate age	Developmental level
3 years 6 months	Children have a wide vocabulary and word usage is usually correct; this continues to increase They are now able to use complete sentences although word order is sometimes incorrect Language can now be used to report on past experiences Incorrect word endings are sometimes used, e.g. *swimmed*, *runned*, *seed*
4 years	Children's vocabulary is now extensive; new words are added regularly Longer and more complex sentences are used; sentences may be joined with *because*, which demonstrates an awareness of causes and relationships Children are able to narrate long stories including the sequence of events Play involves running commentaries The boundaries between fact and fiction are blurred and this is reflected in children's speech Speech is fully intelligible with few, minor incorrect uses Questioning is at its peak. 'When?' is used alongside other questions. By this stage children can usually use language to share, take turns, collaborate, argue, predict what may happen, compare possible alternatives, anticipate, give explanations, justify behaviour, create situations in imaginative play, reflect upon their own feelings and begin to describe how other people feel
5 years	Children have a wide vocabulary and can use it appropriately Vocabulary can include colours, shapes, numbers and common opposites, e.g. big/small, hard/soft Sentences are usually correctly structured although incorrect grammar may still be used Pronunciation may still be childish Language continues to be used and developed as described in the section on 4-year-olds; this may now include phrases heard on the television and associated with children's toys. Questions and discussions are for enquiry and information; questions become more precise as children's cognitive skills develop Children will offer opinions in discussion

APPENDIX C: REFERENCING

Harvard System for references and bibliographies
This form may be photocopied

Organisation of references and bibliography
- All books and publications should be listed in alphabetical order by author.
- If a candidate is using more than one item by the same author the items should be listed in date order.
- For each author single-authored items should be listed first, then joint-authored items and finally multiple-authored items. Within these sections items should be listed in date order. For two or more items by the same author with the same date candidates should label them in the text:
    Syer, W. (1990a)
    Syer, W. (1990b)
  In the references these items would appear as:
    Syer, W (1990a) Children at Play, Children's Education, pp 28-29
    Syer, W (1990b) The Relevance of Comfort, Issues in Child Care, p 13

Organisation of books
- In the assignment: 'Smith (1974) has argued that . . .'
- In the list of references at the end of the assignment (organised as above) 'Smith, P. (1974) Methods of Child Observation, Newton, Hodginson Press'.

Two authors
- In the assignment: 'Biggs and Pool (1976) indicated that . . .'
- In the references: 'Biggs, S and Pool, H (1976) Studies in Child Development, Reading, PUI Press'

Quotations
More than four lines in quotations must be referenced.

© CACHE
from Diploma Assessment Handbook (Appendices)